# A SMILE AT
# *Twilight*

*Enjoy !*

*Robert Loyst*

## ROBERT LOYST &
## WAYNE YETMAN

◆ FriesenPress

Suite 300 - 990 Fort St
Victoria, BC, Canada, V8V 3K2
www.friesenpress.com

Cover image © Stephanie Jermyn Woods

Acknowledgements: Our Curious Comma (hb)

Production Assistant: Heather McDonald

**ISBN**
978-1-4602-6118-7 (Hardcover)
978-1-4602-6119-4 (Paperback)
978-1-4602-6120-0 (eBook)

*1. Family & Relationships, Eldercare*

Distributed to the trade by The Ingram Book Company

# A SMILE AT TWILIGHT

Most stories about Alzheimer's focus on loss.
This one is different.
Within the shadows of receding
friendships and memories,
I was blessed to share time, antics,
and laughter with a woman of
unbridled spirit.
This book contains cherished
recollections of our unlikely friendship.

-Robert Loyst-

# Table of Contents

This is a true story: The names and
some places have been changed.

To Stephanie Jermyn Woods

*My Inspiration*

# The Journey Begins

Have you ever gone to a job interview? Do you remember your nervous stomach, your trembling hands? Well then, you have a good idea how I felt when I pulled into Poppy's driveway on that drab December morning in 2010. It wasn't that I particularly needed a job; I was happily retired, and really just looking for something to keep me busy a few hours a week. If the interview went badly I'd simply go home and find something else.

It wasn't the interview that was bothering me. I was worried about dealing with Poppy herself. I'd heard so many stories about her domineering ways, and how each and every assistant who had been on the scene so far had either quit (usually) or been fired (occasionally) within days of starting. Poppy was apparently so demanding that few (perhaps no one) could live up to her expectations. Would she blast me out of the water in our first encounter?

I sat in the car for several minutes, trying to collect myself. Driving down through Rosedale always made me jumpy. It's so easy to get lost. Many of the streets don't make sense. In fact, most of them aren't really streets at all. They're crescents or squares or closes or circles, or at the very least avenues or drives. They twist and turn and double back on each other, peter out, appear to end, then abruptly start up again a block or so this way or the other. It's like a maze. And that morning that confusion seemed to perfectly match my situation. I really didn't know what I was getting myself into.

But I'm an optimist. I told myself there was no point in getting down at the mouth. A stint in Rosedale is hardly the end of the world. It would be fun to see how the wealthy have chosen to spend their money. Like it or not, their sprawling stone mansions with the lush gardens and stately Georgian piles hidden behind brick walls, and the massive, broad-beamed Tudor homes pretending to be rustic cottages all offer a glimpse of what it's like to be rich in Toronto. Every home is different, yet every home seems to speak the same language. That language is money. And this was to be my territory for the next couple of years. Rosedale was Poppy country. And there I was, ready or not.

I took a deep breath and got out of the car. *In for a penny, in for a pound,* I said to myself.

I suppose I'm basically an idealist. Poppy had a problem – she had been diagnosed with the initial stages of Alzheimer's disease. Surely, that was reason enough to cut her a little slack. Perhaps the people around her weren't allowing for how that disease can affect normal behaviour. Maybe I could be the one to cut through all that and help her enjoy her life a little bit more. Alternatively, maybe I was being foolish, rushing in where a wiser man might just say, "Hold on, I've got enough headaches already. Let's just think about this a little more."

I knew she had money so her house in Rosedale merely confirmed it. It was a stately Georgian with what seemed like a mile of manicured lawn in front and it had an imposing burgundy door with gleaming copper hardware. Intimidating, in other words.

I rang the bell, waited a long minute, and then knocked. A few more seconds and the door opened. A handsome Doberman slipped out to greet me. I had been advised to expect a dog so this didn't bother me a bit. I'd had a Doberman of my own years ago. I felt his cold nose on my hand as he gave me the usual sniff test. Being a dog lover, I continued to carry dog treats, so I intuitively reached into my pocket and offered him a couple of biscuits. To me this casual gesture was simply the normal way to greet man's best friend. However, as it happened, it changed everything.

A slim, older woman with a pleasant smile stepped forward and extended her hand. It was a very firm hand-shake. She was wearing a pair of brown slacks and a simple beige blouse. I'd been told she was eighty years old but she didn't look it. She wore little if any makeup and she didn't seem to need it. "I'm Poppy," she said. "This is Prince. We should go to the living room."

Her voice was hardly menacing. In fact, she sounded friendly. The dog marched ahead and Poppy and I followed.

Jane, the young social worker who had coached me on how to behave around Poppy, was already sitting there. She smiled nervously. This was a test for both of us. I knew she didn't want to fail yet again.

It was an elegant living room with early-American antiques and a beige chesterfield. There were two chairs positioned in front of the window with their backs to a formal garden. Jane was sitting in one of them and I took Poppy's direction and sat in the other. Poppy took a seat off to the side, angled so that she was facing us but towards the window. An interrogation seemed imminent.

Poppy sat back, apparently leaving it to us to justify our presence. Prince made the first move. Before anyone could say anything, he pounced on a tennis ball lying on the floor and thrust it into my lap. It wasn't quite the normal way to start a job interview, but I grabbed the soppy thing and sent it bouncing across the carpet.

Prince leapt after it and was back in an instant. This time, I sent it rolling down the hallway and we all automatically watched the dog as he chased it down and came roaring back.

"Oh, that's so nice to see," said Poppy.

"I used to have a Doberman. They're wonderful. How old is Prince?" I asked.

Poppy smiled and said, "Six years. He's the second one I've had; he is the best."

"My old dog could have been Prince's twin."

I suppose I was expecting to see some immediate evidence of dementia, or at least some of the nasty behaviour that had caused all the problems, but she wasn't unpleasant at all. One might even say, overly polite. I was tempted to ask if I was in the wrong house. Fortunately, I stifled that thought.

We talked about Prince for ten minutes or so. Then Poppy interrupted to ask me to tell her a little about myself. I quickly related how I'd been a chauffeur at Jasper Park Lodge during my student days and had been an avid driver ever since. I said that I'd been in the graphic arts business in Toronto most of my working life; that I'd travelled internationally for my company, at one point as export manager; and that I'd spent five years in South America before returning home to Toronto. I had retired recently, and at my wife's suggestion had contacted the "Seniors Helping Seniors" organization about doing a little work for them. They had suggested that I meet with her.

All of that seemed acceptable, and with those niceties over, we got back to the serious business of admiring Prince.

After a few more minutes Poppy stood up, the interview apparently over. She glanced at Jane, who had been noticeably silent so far.

"Well Poppy?" Jane said.

Poppy gave a bit of a nod and held out her hand to me. "I'll see you tomorrow?"

"I'll phone you tomorrow morning to set up a time," I replied.

"How is two-thirty?"

I groaned inwardly. Two-thirty in the afternoon seemed like an awful time to be fighting Toronto traffic, even in genteel Rosedale. Nevertheless, that could be resolved later. "I'll be here."

As Poppy and Prince turned to lead us out, I glanced at Jane. She lifted her eyes and gave me a surreptitious thumbs-up sign. My guess was that she was thrilled I had passed the first test, and felt that this at least would delay the next disaster. The entire visit had taken a little less than half an hour.

Playing with the dog seemed to have been the key. Poppy's attitude appeared to have been that if you're good enough for my dog, then you're good enough for me.

She said good-bye at the door. She was neither warm nor cold, but efficiently polite. She had the situation well under control.

A discussion about why I was there never arose. There was no mention of Alzheimer's or her situation – nothing about why she needed an aide. The rules of engagement or expectations never entered the conversation. I knew little more when I left than when I had arrived, except that I had landed the job.

My wife, Stephanie, was sitting in the living room when I got home. She looked up, her eyes bright, "Well?" she said.

I paused before I answered. I wasn't quite sure what to say. "I start tomorrow. But I don't know whether I'm riding a bronco or a pony – she's a hard one to read."

Stephanie chuckled. "Just your cup of tea."

I smiled weakly. I really had no idea what lay ahead. But I suspected it would be a lot more than it first appeared.

***

# Robert

My name is Robert. I'm seventy years old but people say I don't look it. I have ailments, yes, but overall I'm pretty fit. I have a goodly head of silver hair, but again, people say I look young for my age. They could be lying but I don't argue. If Poppy was supposed to be hot-tempered, I'm the polar opposite. It takes a lot to get me riled up.

I lost my mother when I was eight and was brought up by my Aunt Catherine. She taught me that making enemies wasn't the way to find happiness in life. "Stay calm," she used to say. "Stay calm and you won't grate on people." I've never regretted taking her advice.

Let me start by offering you some disclaimers: I'm not a doctor. Nor am I a writer. You can't rely on me for subtle explanations about Alzheimer's and dementia. I suppose there is a difference between the two, but I'm not entirely clear what it might be. On the surface, it didn't really matter when we launched into all this. I was to be Poppy's aide, not her caregiver. I am neither a psychologist nor a psychiatrist. I won't be able to wow you with complex explanations of her symptoms, nor will I rhapsodize about the profound implications of all that happened between Poppy and me. I don't want to misrepresent myself. I'll simply tell you my story, and you can judge for yourself.

I spent almost my entire career in sales. I know what it's like to invest weeks of time in cultivating a new client and then get turned down. I know about those late-day calls where a long time (and lucrative) customer tells you he's found someone cheaper and you're off the job. I know what it's like to deal with surly executives and angry workmen.

I guess I pride myself on my ability to manage unpleasant situations and nasty people. It's simply the way I am.

Poppy, as I would quickly see, was at war, or at the very least at a tenuous stalemate, with most (if not all) of the people who were trying to help her. For some reason she and I were to take off on a journey that neither of us could have predicted. It was to be a perilous trip, with many challenges, but along the way we were to lead each other on a merry chase, and I would learn a lot more about Poppy and dealing with Alzheimer's and dementia – more than I could have ever imagined. I'd also discover how important the miracle of human communication is to all of us.

Since I am telling you my story, I obviously must feel that I gained something from my experience with Poppy.

I hope that I can share some insights that might resonate with a loved one coping with someone suffering through this dreadful disease. Indeed, I hope for more than that.

I hope to entertain you a little, since life with Poppy was certainly not maudlin. Poppy drove me crazy, she tested my patience, she tried my people skills, and she challenged my 'grace under pressure.'

Poppy was an extraordinary woman. She was a singular individual who had grown up in unusual circumstances, developed a steel-like independent streak, and was lucky enough to have the financial resources to push that independence to the limit.

She was proud, intelligent, beautiful, and strong; occasionally her wilfulness would erupt in anger. The traits that guided her through her early life did not evaporate when the Alzheimer's began. Poppy was always Poppy.

***

# The Driving Day

The morning after my interview, I phoned Poppy at ten a.m. She answered. I would later observe that she was always the only one in the house who answered the phone. In fact, she made it abundantly clear to anyone there that it was her phone and she alone would answer it. That was the law.

"Hi Poppy, it's Robert. Just wanted to confirm our meeting."

"How is two-thirty?"

"Fine. I'll see you then."

You'll notice I called her Poppy right from the start. She had introduced herself that way and I simply followed her lead. I never once called her by her full name. It never came up as an issue. It just happened.

Poppy and Prince both came to the door when I knocked. There was a biscuit for Prince, of course; this would become our routine. Poppy beamed with pleasure. I don't think most people realize that getting along with someone's pet is a prerequisite for friendship. Being a dog lover, I know that if your dog likes someone you meet, then you're probably on safe ground.

"Good afternoon," Poppy said. "Just sit down and I'll be right back."

She pointed me to a chair down the hall in the vestibule. Prince bounced after her, but a few seconds later was back again with his ball. The hall was very long so I threw it right down to the end. Prince raced down and was back in a flash. Back and forth, we went several times.

Suddenly Prince changed his mind, sought out his Kong in a corner, and brought it back to me. I was contemplating whether it was safe to send the huge rubber toy spinning down the hall when Poppy reappeared.

"I hope he's not bothering you too much," she said.

I shook my head. Playing with Prince was bringing back memories of my own dogs. However, something in Poppy's voice told me I'd better not go too far with her noble beast. Was she perhaps a little jealous of Prince's new affiliation?

"I have my list," she said.

Little did I know how that list would come to rule my life.

There were sixteen coats in the closet; everything from a summer-light windbreaker to Arctic-worthy parkas. She asked me about the weather, and then selected the one she wanted. I helped her on with it, but I sensed she was only reluctantly accepting my assistance. It was probably the first hint of her fierce resistance to relinquishing control over any decision whatsoever. By the way, I didn't think that her slowness in choosing her coat was a symptom of dementia — it merely struck me as the price of having so many coats.

Maybe not.

By the time, we got outside and she was ensconced in the passenger side of my old car, she hadn't said anything about our destination.

"Where are we off to, Poppy?"

"I'll show you how to get there when we're out in the street. I don't know the street names but I know how to get there."

As we came out of the circular drive, the directions began.

"Go along here. Left here," she said a few minutes later. "Right here."

We worked our way down to Carlton where she directed me into the right-hand lane and then abruptly told me to pull over and stop. I obeyed, wondering what we were doing. She jumped out and leaned over as she closed the door. "You wait here. I'll be back," she said.

I watched her march into the pet store. Then I waited and waited. What was she doing that could take so long? Twenty minutes later, she was back to the car, with a bag full of tins of cat food. I wanted to open the door for her, but she was sitting beside me before I could move.

"Everything OK?" I asked.

She glanced at me as if I was a vagrant seeking a handout, and waved her hand at the windshield. "Straight ahead... Turn left...Turn down there."

With her giving the orders and me obeying, we made our way to a shoe repair store, a hardware store, a drug store, then a convenience store. She clearly had a plan and just as clearly wasn't going to share it with me. It was a tad frustrating not knowing where we were going, but I tried to see it from her point of view. She was probably used to driving to these places herself. It must be frustrating describing it to a driver rather than just doing it yourself.

We got home about five-thirty. It was dark and the traffic was at its height as people left their offices to head home. She let herself out of the car and announced: "Just sit there; call me tomorrow."

She grabbed the parcels and made for her front door. Apparently, I had passed the test. I would have walked her to the door, but she got out so fast it was impossible. I was already sensing that kind of helpful conduct was unnecessary and would be an annoyance to her.

I was right. Later on in our adventures, I got out several times to help and she immediately reminded me that she was quite capable of opening the door and didn't need any assistance. I'm an old-fashioned type of person – I think anyone watching would think less of me if I didn't help a woman out of a car. I overcame that inhibition quickly.

If Poppy wanted a modern guy, then I would be her man.

On the way home, I couldn't help chuckling. I suppose
I should have been insulted that she wouldn't even let me
know where we were going. Nevertheless, something about
her reminded me of my late aunt who had brought me
up. She had been a soft-spoken but no-nonsense woman
who knew exactly what she wanted and quietly made sure
it happened. It seemed to me she had been resurrected in
Poppy's form.

\*\*\*

# Looking For A Job

Several months before I encountered Poppy I was retired and bored. Stephanie, my wife, saw some ads on TV for the local organization, "Seniors Helping Seniors." It appeared to offer a number of services for older people and Stephanie, seeing me at loose ends, suggested that I see if they would employ me.

So one morning I made my way over to their Toronto offices on St. Clair at Yonge Street.

No. They weren't hiring. The young woman behind the counter suggested I call in the spring. I shrugged and headed for the door. She called me back.

"Wait a minute," she said. "You're not a bad looking guy. We have a client who has rejected everyone we've sent. You could be our last hope."

Not a bad looking guy? People seem to say the most ridiculous things to seniors. In this case, she was obviously very discerning.

"Nothing ventured, nothing gained," I said. The warning about what lay ahead was lost on me. Not a bad looking guy? I was putty in her hands.

"Why don't you fill in an application?"

I completed it on the spot. I put in references, and they were impressed to see that a nun was one of those supporting me. I suppose they checked those references because they called me back soon after.

First, there was an interview with Myra, one of the owners of "Seniors Helping Seniors." She asked me right off if I was prepared to deal with an extremely difficult person. She said everyone they had sent to Poppy had been rejected or had quit. They complained that the woman in question was a nasty and impossible person. Some of their staff weren't even making it through the interview with the client, and Myra saw her as a challenge. What else could I do but assure her I would try my best?

Then, one of Myra's staff, Rosemary, spoke to me – more of the same: "Do you think you can cope?"

I didn't know what to think. How could one woman cause such problems? Even if she was such a horror, what could that really mean to an assistant? I mean, my role, ostensibly, was to help her with her life. How much trouble can you get into doing that?

Next, I met the social worker, Jane, in a little coffee shop just across from the office on St. Clair. Jane was a charming young woman in her mid-twenties; good looking, cute in a daughterly way, and very bubbly.

"What would you do if our client started an argument with you?" Jane asked.

"I suppose I'd agree with her," I said, "and try to change the subject. If she persisted then I'd try to say as little as possible. Let her vent her point of view. That's Sales 101."

"What if she won't do what you want her to do some day? Perhaps, a minor request, like, please get in the car. What would you do if she simply refused?"

"Oh, I think I would just go along with it. Why argue? I'd offer to take her for a walk instead. Really, I'd do whatever she wants. Let her be the boss. Let her have her way. As long as she isn't in danger, what's the point of me trying to force her to do anything? After all, I work for her. She doesn't work for me."

"What will you do if she starts swearing at you?"

I grinned. The old woman was going to swear at me? Wow. She certainly sounded like a tiger. "Well I don't care what she calls me. I'm old enough to have heard just about everything. I suspect I'd be tempted to laugh, but that likely wouldn't be a good idea. I'd probably just let her go on, knowing she would come back to earth eventually."

Jane wanted to know if I got along with animals. Their client apparently had not only a huge Doberman but also a big and unsociable Siamese cat. By this point, she was smiling. I sensed some relief. Apparently, she had found someone who just might pass the test.

"I'd like you to meet our client," she finally said. "Her name is Poppy. You two just might get along."

"I'll give it a whirl."

"Please. We've tried our best and she's impossible."

Finally!

I had a telephone interview with Anna, Poppy's daughter, who lived in Utica, NY. Anna was even more to the point than all the other people with whom I had spoken. Her mother, she told me, could be controlling, demanding, and precise in what she wanted. "Her likes and dislikes will be very clear," she said, "yet she won't want to discuss why." Anna struck me as articulate and down to earth. As time went by, her candid assessment of her mother was to prove very accurate.

"Do you have any experience with these kinds of people?" she asked.

"It's pretty difficult to say when you've never met the person," I answered. "My mother-in-law had Alzheimer's and several other family members haven't exactly been angels. I can appreciate where you're coming from."

Underneath her blunt assessment, I could tell that Anna was a loving daughter striving to ensure the best care for her mother. She wanted me to email her after a week to report how things were going. I heard an unspoken message in her voice: *If you last a week.*

I spoke by telephone as well with Edward, one of Poppy's
sons who lived in Hartford, Connecticut. He was less busi-
ness-like than Anna and talked with a smile in his voice. I
found his perception of his mother fascinating.

"My mother is different. She can be aloof, as well as a bit
of a know-it-all. Other than that, she's reasonably likeable.
You probably heard more details from my sister."

I explained what Anna had said, and he laughed. "It's not
all that bad."

Edward seemed to be somewhat more at ease with his
mother than Anna − a light-hearted person. Anna was
charming but not as carefree.

"Be flexible," Edward said. "She may ask you to do anything. She's an off-the-wall person who gets something in
her mind and won't rest until it's the way she wants it."

I felt more comfortable after talking to Edward. There
might be hope. But Anna's point of view did weigh on me.
Was she being overly pessimistic or simply more realistic?

Through all of this, I could see that as much as they
were checking my suitability as Poppy's aide, they were really
more concerned about my ability to deal with their mother
than with her getting along with me. I admit it was unset-
tling. She had a dreadful reputation.

Nevertheless, like Anna, Edward seemed to be content
with what I had to offer and sent me on my way with a positive feeling.

"Good luck and please keep in touch."

24    So there I was – fully approved and ready to meet the challenge. After all this build-up, I figured the chances of Poppy and me getting along were about fifty/fifty. I was expecting the worst…that I wouldn't prove good enough for her. It appeared that nobody was able to satisfy her. Keep in mind; I was the fifth candidate to try out. The two children had given me different pictures of their mother with the only common thread being that she was incredibly difficult. It was confusing but I tried not to think about it.

Let the chips fall where they may.

***

# Poppy's Routine

Our first few weeks passed much like the first day. I phoned
– Poppy told me when to arrive. After dealing with her mail,
appointments, pills, etc., we ran errands.

She told me where to turn and where to stop. She
shopped – I waited. She finished – I drove her home. Then
– do it again the next day. Then the day after that, and the
next day, and again, and again.

I found her intimidating. I felt like I was walking on
tissue paper. She was almost impossible to read; she gave
me no indication of what she liked or disliked; no reaction
– nothing. She was very much in control. To my mind, if she
did have Alzheimer's then on a scale of one to ten, she must
have been at one. I learned from talking with her friends and
family that she had always been very blunt and straightforward, and that the Alzheimer's had merely exaggerated this

behaviour. She knew exactly what she wanted and she knew that she was right.

I was most concerned with making sure she found me compatible. It was very strange. Knowing the situation, I didn't find her difficult, but I could see that if anyone had walked in cold and tried to be jolly or all-controlling, this would have created a confrontational situation.

I kept my ears open and my mouth shut.

She seemed to appreciate that. She never really chatted. In fact, I'd have to say she hated chatting. She was polite; she had all the graces. However, simply talking for the sake of talking, of passing the time by commenting on the weather or some minor incident was obviously unacceptable to her sensibilities.

She rarely said thank you. In a peculiar circumstance, she might say; "You don't have to do that," but not, 'thank you.' However, everything she did say seemed sincere. She simply didn't appear to like saying 'sorry' or 'please' or 'thank you' casually. She did not throw those words around the way many of us do.

She might say, "Would you mind?" That was her way of saying, 'please.'

The whole time I worked for Poppy, we never really had a lengthy conversation. She often wanted my opinion, but not a discussion on any given matter. She liked things to be cut and dried – black and white.

That struck me as strange at first. She was well educated and well read. She was intelligent. She had travelled extensively. Why was she so reticent in conversation? The answer only came to me much later. Despite her forceful personality and her cherished independence, her memory was fading. It wasn't that she chose not to engage in conversations, I suspect she simply wasn't capable of engaging with anyone for any length of time.

Soon after I had met her, I recognized that with Poppy it was better not to say anything unless I really had something to say. I found it better all-around to let her come to me. The result was that we'd sit in silence much of the time. Every so often, she observed something out the window of the car.

"Look at that," she said.

"Oh yes. Very interesting," I replied.

That was it. She seemed content to hear "very interesting." It almost became a kind of code. It meant that I had heard her and understood her. That was all she seemed to need or want. The fact that I was often so distracted with the traffic that I didn't know what she was talking about didn't matter at all. "Very interesting" did the trick.

My old car was a bit of an embarrassment. I shared it with my daughter, who is a veterinarian, and has three cats and a dog. To me it smelled like an animal clinic. Poppy hadn't shown any trace of noticing it, but after a week or so, I suggested she might be more comfortable in her own car.

"Fine," she said. That was it. I drove her in her own Mercedes from that point on. She didn't seem to care one way or the other, but I enjoyed the step up in luxury.

28 Poppy was a perfectionist. I'm more of a take-it-as-it-comes type of guy. However, for her everything had to be just so except, oddly, the car. It could be relatively dirty, but the windows had to be immaculately clean. I made a point of checking when I arrived. She wanted to see out perfectly. When it was threatening rain, after the first drops, she said: "Aren't you going to turn on the windshield wipers?"

Poppy may have been reluctant to chat, but she certainly knew how to swear. I wasn't with her long before "shit" and "Jesus Christ" emerged as expressions of her indignation. It unnerved me at first, because I was already in fear of her, and these expletives from a woman jarred me further. Funny though, her swearing always seemed to fit the situation. Nevertheless, it didn't take long for me to accept these profanities as part of her conversation and to let them fade into the scenery.

I wondered where she could have picked up such a vocabulary. She was articulate and refined in almost everything she said, except when these profanities rushed to the fore.

Then there was the 'glare.' When she saw or heard something contrary to her wishes, Poppy had a glare that would wither a flagpole. Her eyes narrowed, her cheek twitched ever so slightly, and she leaned forward into your face just enough to give you the impression that she was inspecting the bottom of the toilet bowl. That glare was an awesome penalty to endure and I did everything I could to avoid it.

You are probably assuming that such a woman was hugely argumentative. Not at all. Poppy rarely argued. More precisely, she demanded. She would never ask what we were going to do next. She knew exactly what she wanted to do next. Did she need my ideas? No. If I wanted to do something else, well then, that really wasn't going to happen.

"Well Poppy, where do you want to go?"

"Pet store."

"Anywhere else?"

"I'll tell you when we're finished there."

Despite these eccentricities, Poppy seemed happy. She was living her way. She devoted her days to a raft of domestic duties that appeared to add up to a lot of pleasure. She loved eating and put a lot of effort into planning her meals. She liked going out in the car, but only for a specific destination, never for a recreational drive. She considered that a waste of time. At first, we went out four times a week.

After a while, it grew to five. Sometimes our errands took most of the afternoon, and sometimes just a couple of hours. Despite her reluctance to let me in on her daily plan of attack, she seemed to bask in the thrill of the purchase.

Poppy walked Prince in the nearby park every morning and evening, and as best I could tell, she had many dog-loving friends there and enjoyed seeing them. She had a Siamese cat that she doted on, reserving its feeding and the emptying of the litter box exclusively to herself.

She enjoyed her home and closely supervised the cleaning lady to ensure everything was the way she wanted it. She spent a lot of time at her desk, writing cheques to the many charities that sought to profit from her affection for animals. Strangely, her home was tidy and well organized, while her private office and desk were chaotic, something which made organizing her much more difficult.

Her daughter Anna called virtually every day, and her good friend Mary Johnston often called from the U.S.A.

Her den, just off the dining room, had floor-to-ceiling bookcases, like a library. The book collection was extensive, mainly European and African history and political books. She wasn't interested in frivolous reading; there were no romances or thrillers. She'd been all over the world, and had obviously spent a lot of time pondering her place in that world. She read the *Globe and Mail* newspaper every morning, as well as the *New York Times* on weekends.

Every Tuesday I drove her to her badminton lessons at the Granite Club, and Thursdays we went for her exercise class. The personal trainer there told me she was very athletic for someone her age and especially talented at badminton. However, every time I brought her home, she would complain about how the exercise classes were too easy and boring. She felt she was wasting her time. I talked to the trainer several times to see what she could do, but she said she didn't want to strain Poppy and didn't know what to do.

Over the course of a few months, I started arriving earlier until we were going out at 10:30 a.m. That was a lot more pleasant for traffic and tied in nicely with our daily trips to

the local supermarket. Poppy ate only fresh food so we had    31
to shop for groceries every day.

At first I drove quite slowly as I wasn't quite sure how she wanted me to behave behind the wheel. I was very careful and made sure I obeyed all the rules of the road. I soon learned that such attention to safety annoyed her.

She obviously had not driven that way herself.

She criticized my driving only twice. She announced that I was too nice to other drivers and I should speed it up a bit. "It's not necessary to stop at the stop signs in Rosedale," she said, "unless someone is coming. It's a waste of time."

That was a bit much to swallow. I mean, I had the driver's licence, not her. I was hesitant to speak up, but I knew that it was important for me to take a bit of a stand on this issue.

"Poppy," I said, "if I lose my license, then neither one of us can drive."

She cocked her head and regarded me with narrowed eyes for several seconds. It was almost 'the glare.' Then it faded.

"OK."

I was shocked. She who ruled all had accepted my comment as a logical reason for stopping at the stop signs. "OK" seemed to be almost like, "Well, you got me." For the first time her single mindedness had been breached. Even if she had Alzheimer's, she was still able to distinguish logic.

She may have been stubborn, but she wasn't stupid.

This kind of event confused me. On the one hand, I really couldn't see many signs of her illness. She was so strong and decisive that it seemed improbable to me that her mind was giving way. She was running her household successfully and setting the agenda for everything she touched. Her behaviour didn't appear to be that of someone who was suffering from Alzheimer's.

On the other hand, perhaps I was (and am) fooling myself. There were certainly hints, yes. She had endless trouble with the TV remote. (But don't we all?)

The neighbours regaled me with stories about her previous social life and the wonderful dinner parties she used to host with the finest gourmet foods, fascinating guests, and inspired conversation.

There were pictures around the house of Poppy dressed in gorgeous gowns at the ballet or the opera. In family albums, I found shots of her dressed very nicely indeed; casual, dressy, and expensive. She appeared to be in her element. In many of the shots, she was clearly in some exotic part of the world.

That reality was history. There were no parties now, and very few nights on the town. The fact was that the invitations had stopped. I suppose that when the word gets around that you have dementia, people start to assume that you can no longer interact normally. Perhaps they feel they might feel uncomfortable in your company. Whatever, her old crowd had pretty well evaporated. Occasionally she would invite a friend over, but nothing that would take much effort.

The beautiful clothing had disappeared as well. During the entire time I was with her, I don't think I saw her in a

skirt more than two or three times. She mostly wore a
blouse and a pair of slacks, always in neutral colours, nothing
splashy. She dressed much the same every day. In hindsight, I
suppose that made life easier for her. She didn't have to think
very much about what top went with what pair of pants. I
don't remember if I really considered that at the time.

She rarely mentioned her past life. I suppose that was an
indicator of dementia, but if it was, it took a long time for me
to catch on. I sometimes wondered if she realized something
was wrong and was gamely attempting to hide it.

Our conversations, brief as they were, rarely went in that
direction, and so be it. She never mentioned Alzheimer's in
the whole time I knew her.

One day I asked her why she couldn't drive.

"I was seeing the psychiatrist and he told me I couldn't
drive anymore," she said.

"I'm sorry," I said. "That's too bad."

"So am I. I can't drive, so I don't drive."

That was Poppy to a tee. She had a practical way of
dealing with reality. She would fight the changeable, but if it
were obvious that a situation was beyond change, she simply
accepted that and moved on. She was not one for moaning
and groaning about life's misfortunes. Maybe a few expletives to vent her frustration, and then off she went.

Despite these hints of problems, Poppy was still one of
the most interesting people I had ever met. I was so busy
trying to get along and understand her; I rarely saw anything
beyond her lifestyle and temperament.

I couldn't see very much wrong with her. She certainly could, on occasion, forget about another person's feelings, but she was always more or less good to me.

The important thing was that we got along so well. With some people, you just immediately find a connection. I drifted into enjoying her company. I think I mentioned earlier that I had worked in sales most of my career. Well, dealing with Poppy neatly dovetailed with many of the skills I had picked up in my working life. I had always had an instinctive feel for when clients wanted me to explain things in detail or when they wanted me to keep quiet while they thought things through. I was used to being turned down but still calmly persevering until something clicked and I got the sale.

I remember quaffing beer in pubs with workmen on whom I depended to make my product work, and I remember sitting in a gorgeous boardroom listening to a self-important CEO try to cajole me into cutting my price just a little bit more.

Everyone is different. Everyone has his or her own quirks and mannerisms. I learned not to fight human nature. It works a lot better if you accept people as they are and try to manage things so everyone gets something he or she wants.

So it was with Poppy. All her habits, her unusual mannerisms, her colourful vocabulary – none of it bothered me. It was simply Poppy being Poppy, and I liked her. She had a lovely voice, always very clear and more than occasionally embarrassingly louder than necessary.

Where does the job begin and where does it end? Poppy
was sort of fun. She was interesting. Life in her presence was
not dull. There was always an air of anticipation; something
of interest was always going to happen.

I'd say we coasted along that way for almost a year. If
the Alzheimer's was making progress, it was hard to see.
Sometimes I would look back at the end of a month and ask
myself if anything had changed. Usually the answer was no.
It was so small, such a gradual thing. Not to worry.

***

# Marlena Lang (a.k.a. Poppy)

Why did this woman called Poppy need me? The polite answer, and the answer I'd been given when I first appeared in Poppy's life, was that a psychiatrist had forbidden her to drive anymore. In the initial part of our relationship, taking over the driving turned out to be a bigger part of my job than managing her daily activities. Apparently, she was in an early stage of Alzheimer's and the doctor thought it safest to take away her driving licence.

The less polite answer, as I soon learned from her friends, was that she was a holy terror on the roads. One of her friends told me that she had driven with Poppy once and would never do it again. Another said that driving with Poppy had 'tested her mettle.' Whether Poppy's aggressive driving was a symptom of Alzheimer's or simply part of her personality puzzled me at first. However, as I learned a little more about her history, I came to suspect that Poppy's behind-the-wheel behaviour was more a part of her character than a result of her disease. You will hear me say this more than a few times in the course of this story. Poppy was not what I first envisioned her to be as an individual or a passenger.

As I've said, she rarely said much about herself. But through talking with her daughter and the neighbours, I gradually pieced together a little bit of her history. She had grown up on a farm in northern Maine. Her grandfather had started the farm, eking out a difficult existence on the rocky soil, assisted later by his son, Poppy's father. Her father died young, and while her mother worked in New York as a nurse, Poppy lived on the farm with her grandparents.

It was a difficult life, but Poppy apparently thrived on it. One story is that her mother came to visit her, and in Poppy's enthusiasm about farm life, she let loose a series of colourful phrases to describe how farm animals reproduce that left her mother shocked. That was the end of the farm scene for Poppy. She was packed off to a series of private boarding schools.

I say a series of schools because apparently, she was a bit of a hellion and more than a number of these lofty institutions had bargained for. I am leading you astray here, because I imagine you'd like to know more about what she did and how it provoked a constant change of address. The truth is I have no idea. Poppy rarely talked about herself and even less about her schooling. She might have been hiding some dark and dangerous secret of course, but I think otherwise. It simply wasn't part of Poppy's nature to talk about herself. She was very matter of fact. If something needed saying, fine, say it. Poppy, I think, would have seen little importance in her school days and related antics.

Once when we went shopping together, I suggested that we might buy some cauliflower. "Don't talk to me about cauliflower," she said. "I ate far too much of that vile stuff in boarding school." This was more or less the extent of her schooldays revelations.

Poppy was intelligent and had studied horticulture at Cornell. This was the beginning of a life-long fascination with gardening. She also studied languages, could speak fluent French, and her command of German was extensive. She had developed good writing skills, and became interested in animal husbandry.

Details of her life after graduation from Cornell were just as sketchy as they were for her earlier schooling. Poppy was reluctant to discuss her past, and anything she did reveal was usually very brief. For example, we saw a motorcycle one day while out doing errands, and she casually mentioned that she and a girlfriend had gone out to Vancouver on the backs of motorcycles with some guys. The girls dropped the guys and ended up independent in Vancouver.

End of story.

Nothing more. It was as if a memory had surfaced for a moment, then had fled the scene as quickly as it had arrived. Was it the dementia or simply her quest for privacy? Despite the natural inclination to blame her idiosyncrasies on Alzheimer's, the truth was more difficult to determine. The more I knew her, the more she revealed her real personality, which overshadowed her disease.

There is nothing to indicate she ever worked for money. Her maiden name, by the way, was Lang – Marlena Lang. No one seems to know how she got the nickname Poppy but it stuck. Everyone I ever met called her Poppy, not Marlena.

In her late twenties, Poppy married Walter Henkel. Shortly thereafter their three children – Edward, George, and Anna were born. Henkel was an outstanding business-man. It was his money that sustained Poppy's demand-ing lifestyle.

When Poppy did occasionally mention her family, it was always regarding her children. Her son George was a doctor living in Atlanta. He seemed to have the least involvement with Poppy of any of the children. I never met him. I do though remember one day when Poppy cut her finger and the bleeding seemed to be more than you would expect from a minor wound, that I humorously suggested calling George. It seemed to me that as a doctor he would know something about stopping bleeding.

"No, he's not that kind of doctor; all he does is cut people up," she said.

Anna, down in Utica, was Poppy's only daughter. She was a friendly and attractive woman who managed mul-tiple local charities, competed in marathons and tennis, and often won. My main contact with the family, she was a no-nonsense type, like her mother. Poppy once told me that Anna could be anything she wanted to be.

Anna was a strong-willed individual (just like her mother) and clearly felt that masterminding her mother's situation was her responsibility. I admired her resolve because managing Poppy was like trying to herd mice.

Edward was an insurance executive in Hartford. To me he seemed to play the "good cop" role, as opposed to Anna's "bad cop." In the end, they both played a role in the drama of Poppy's life.

When Poppy and her husband Walter had come to Toronto, they settled in their large home in Rosedale. Anna studied at Havergal College, a private girls' school. The boys went to Crescent School. Walter drowned in a boating accident at their summer home about four years after arriving in Toronto.

After Walter's death, Poppy returned to school. She took some courses at the University of Toronto. She studied medieval history and successfully wrote the exams. Once I stumbled on several of her papers. They were very sophisticated and revolved around the complexities of the economic structure in the fifteenth century. The lowest mark I saw was an A minus, and most of them were A plus.

Poppy was reluctant to discuss her marriage or her education in any detail. One Sunday, on our way to our daily shopping at Summerhill Market, we were driving up Glen Road past the church at Roxborough Road. We had a little perennial joke that we had to get ahead of the church people because a lot of them would end up crowding our market after the service. I took advantage of this to ask her what her religion was.

"Lutheran."

"Do you go to church often?" I asked.

"No, no. I had enough religion in school to last me two lifetimes."

Again, that was it.

With Poppy, you could talk all you wanted and she would respond as long as you had something interesting to say. She wouldn't put up with idle chitchat. She'd rather sit quietly and think her own thoughts. I had the impression that she could look back on a life well lived. From her start as a relatively poor farm girl, she had ended up a wealthy woman in elite Rosedale. She was well educated, and had three highly successful children and a series of pets that she adored.

Music filled her life. She was a regular at the opera, ballet, or any other musical event. I was told she could discuss the performances in detail, commenting on them from the perspective of her own vast experience. She had been very active socially. She loved to entertain, hosting lavish gatherings at her Highland Avenue mansion that attracted the Rosedale elite for fine food, wines, and esoteric conversation. It must be said that the "Rosedale elite" included the dog-people from the park; a close coterie of canine lovers who met regularly in the park to exercise their dogs and solve the problems of the world.

Poppy was a gourmet cook and often made the entire meal herself for her guests. Her kitchen had all the modern gadgets. When I came on the scene, her kitchen bookshelf held a library of exotic cookbooks from all over the world. She had travelled widely in her day, and I suppose she must have collected these during her travels.

She loved animals. I had a feeling that animals had always been her best friends. Her father had died young; she saw very little of her mother while at school, and her husband had travelled incessantly. Maybe she felt that the people in her life had somehow let her down. Whatever her motivation, she loved her pets unconditionally and was devoted to them.

An avid birdwatcher, she always had a number of feeders in her back yard and was religious about keeping them properly stocked. She would frequently pause in her daily routine to stand in the living room and watch the birds fly around the garden and over the feeder. It was easy for her to identify the various species, and she studied their habits.

As I have said, Poppy had led a wonderful life, even a charmed life. I wish that I had known her in those earlier days. She would have been a lot of fun. How much she could remember of those days as the Alzheimer's took over is anyone's guess. Nevertheless, life was changing and I seemed to have arrived just when the past was still visible but storm clouds were building on the horizon.

***

# Poppy At Large

I had been with her only about ten days when one morning Poppy announced that she couldn't find her watch. She was upset. This was a big thing. She always had to know the time. Her plan was to pick up the food at the market, and then go out and buy a new watch.

I suggested that we search around the house a bit more. The watch might show up. It was snowing like crazy and I didn't really want to battle the downtown traffic. She couldn't have cared less and insisted that she'd looked everywhere and we had to get the new one immediately. I hoped she would forget while we were grocery shopping, but when she got a bee in her bonnet she wouldn't let it go.

"Well Poppy, where will we go?"

"I know the place but I forget the name. I'll know it when we see it. Drive down to Bloor St. and I'll recognize it."

I was dubious. It was snowing hard and I could hardly see. The traffic was awful but that proved to be an advantage, as we had to drive slowly so that she could peer out at each building as we passed. We drove a long way along Bloor St. and she was getting increasingly frustrated. Suddenly, she pointed. There it was: The posh Birks jewellery store on the southeast corner of Bay and Bloor.

It was impossible to park, so she told me to let her out and keep driving around the block until she came out again. She pointed at the corner where I should stop to meet her. I really didn't like leaving her on her own, but she was adamant.

Despite her age, Poppy ploughed through the snow bank and disappeared into Birks. I continued up Bay Street and began circling the block. Traffic was so bad that it took me ten minutes to get around once. She wasn't at the appointed meeting spot so I went around again, and then again.

Finally, on the fourth circuit I spotted her at the entrance. I blew the horn, and to my relief she ran down the stairs, manoeuvred through a snow bank, and slipped into the car. She had her new watch, but showed little enthusiasm. She said she had been in a rush and just took the first one that they showed her. Fine. It was a routine sort of watch by my standards, and nothing more was said.

Weeks later Anna called me. She wanted to know about the $2,000 charge from Birks. I was stunned at the price and explained what had happened, trying my best to sound disapproving.

Anna just said, "My God, what will be, will be."

I didn't dare tell Anna that Poppy didn't even like the watch. Poppy never mentioned it again and one day her original watch turned up under a cushion. Poppy thought that it was nice, and that it was good to have a spare. She preferred to wear the new one.

Months later the new watch stopped working, and when I took it back to Birks, they replaced the battery at no charge. The salesperson said it was a very good watch.

"Yes, indeed. Thank you."

Another time, we had a form of instant replay. This time, she couldn't find her sunglasses. She had sunglasses all over the house but we couldn't find any of them and she insisted on a new pair. Immediately, we were off to the Sunglass Hut in Yorkville.

We were there for over an hour, inspecting an endless array of sunglasses ranging in price from $150 to $1,500, to the ones she eventually picked for "only" $300. I thought this was a bargain compared to the $1,500 ones, but I have never spent more than ten dollars on sunglasses.

The funny thing is that Poppy rarely wore sunglasses. She just wanted them. That was the way she was. When she wanted something, then she would buy it, with little concern for price or practicality. She was never arrogant or ostentatious about her purchases. She didn't buy the most expensive item because it was expensive; she didn't buy something cheaper because it was cheaper. If something struck her the right way, then she had to have it. In her mind, this wasn't wasteful. If she liked something, then cost was irrelevant. However, she wouldn't buy anything on sale.

"Look Poppy, there are the butter tarts you like at fifty percent off."

"No. They must be stale."

Discussion closed.

She used to have her knives and scissors sharpened by a roving peddler who drove up and down Highland Avenue. He charged seven dollars to sharpen a pair of scissors. I pointed out to her that we could buy a new pair of scissors for five dollars or less.

"No. The peddler sharpens them properly. A new pair wouldn't work as well."

She was terrible with names. We often met people in the street and she had a good chat with them. As we moved on Poppy turned to me and said, "Who was that?"

"I don't know. She's your friend."

Then she'd laugh. After a while, we developed a system to deal with this problem. When I saw that she was confused, I introduced myself to whoever it was and they in turn introduced themselves to me. Poppy heard their names and then used them in the conversation. We developed this routine because she was well aware of her problem with names and thought our little system worked well. Apparently, she had never been good with names. She knew it. Whether this was Alzheimer's or simply a personal trait wasn't clear to me. I gave her the benefit of the doubt.

Maybe I was in denial.

She never called me 'my aide' or even 'Robert.' She never referred to me as anything. I was just there. I was 'him.' At first, I found this odd until I saw that she called no one by name except for her family. She used 'him,' 'her,' or 'the person across the street,' or 'my friend next door.' Even Emma, who stayed with her several nights a week, or Laura across the street, who had known her for years and was constantly looking in on her, were simply 'her,' or 'the woman across the street.'

One day I happened to be at Poppy's house when the gardener was working in her backyard. It was a very formal French garden – mostly greenery and a few flowers. She could walk out her back door and down a path to a huge birdbath, circle it, and then continue towards a big twelve-foot-high metal artwork with thick stained glass. I once asked her what it was and she told she had seen it in New York and liked it, so she'd had it shipped home. It was very beautiful and definitely arresting.

The gardener was working away and Poppy told him that she wanted some more shrubs. She was very specific about the kind that were required and explained in detail how they were to be cut and picked. She was friendly about it, but assertive at the same time.

Another time she asked me to take her to a garden centre, way out past the airport. It was a long way to travel for some shrubs, but Poppy knew that this centre carried exactly the plants she wanted. She knew which plants she needed, but didn't feel the gardener could be trusted to get them, and she wouldn't settle for less. At the garden centre, she had a wonderful time discussing every little detail with the salesperson. She told him what she wanted and she questioned him on things she wanted clarified. We bought the shrubs, brought them home, and she supervised the gardener planting them just as she had envisaged.

As these adventures played out, I began to observe that she was much more pleasant and accommodating to men than women. She clearly preferred men.

I could see that the same attitude applied to me. It helped that I was a man. She certainly never alluded to it herself, but other people remarked on it to me as well. It's not politically correct to say it, but I sensed that she felt men were smarter than women. Poppy didn't want to talk about baking cookies or arranging tea parties; she preferred world affairs. She felt most women were frivolous and men were more serious.

She didn't care what was happening a block away; she cared about things in Syria or Iraq or some other world-hotspot.

In Poppy's opinion, her upscale neighbourhood was full of women whose best conversations were about each other, the weather, their children, or last week's party. That wasn't Poppy's style. That sounds sexist, doesn't it? Please don't shoot the messenger.

She tried to keep a good distance from these people. Her life had been lived in the company of men and women who were well educated, had significant career responsibilities, and could be counted on to lead a conversation into

challenging topics. For Poppy, men had accomplished a lot    51
more than most women.

The intellectually stimulating days were gone for Poppy
but I was grateful that I was on the right side of her version
of the gender wars. It made my job easier.

*\*\**

# Free Time

You might be wondering how I spent my time when I wasn't with Poppy. Well, that makes for a short chapter.

Poppy, in fact, gradually took over most of my leisure time. I don't think she meant to but as you're seeing, she was relentless in her pursuits. It was go-go-go to keep up with her.

Sometimes I'd get home at the end of the day and Stephanie would simply steer me to a nice stiff scotch.

"A tough one?" she asked.

I groaned. "Tough isn't the word. I love working with her; it's just that she is so active. And I have to be on my guard all the time. I'm somehow responsible for her – but she doesn't want any part of that deal."

Stephanie laughed. "You're an even better man than I thought."

"Thanks. Maybe one day I'll write a book about all this."

But lest you think I'm an old codger who dozed away my time when I wasn't with Poppy, let me say that I have lots of other interests in life. I play chess, do crosswords; I read a lot – non-fiction, histories, and biographies. I love cars and you'll often find me at auto shows or at dealers. I like seeing the latest prototypes and analyzing their pros and cons.

I also do some on and off consulting work. I have a client in China whose English isn't very good so he uses me to make initial contacts here in Canada. Sometimes I accompany him when he meets Canadian clients to make sure they understand what he is proposing.

Do you believe all this? I'm afraid I'm stretching the truth a wee bit. There is no escaping that Poppy really occupied a huge part of my life for a prolonged period. Despite a little bit of moaning and groaning when I got home to Steph…it was exhilarating.

\*\*\*

# The First Christmas

Let me confess that at my age Christmas doesn't quite grab me the way it used to. Call me Scrooge, but all the bother sometimes doesn't seem worth it. So, after two weeks on the job with Poppy, the sudden dash to Christmas not only brought a whole new level of challenge to my life but also eradicated my complacency about Poppy and Alzheimer's.

A Christmas tree was her first priority. Poppy had to have a Christmas tree. Poppy, in fact, had to have a very specific Christmas tree. As I was coming to understand, she was a perfectionist. She knew exactly what tree she wanted and how it had to look – a certain species, a certain shape, and above all, big, big, big.

Unfortunately, Poppy had the vision but the world didn't seem willing to co-operate, at least in her mind. One day we went off in the car on a grand tour of Christmas tree lots. I had never realized how many Christmas tree dealers appear on the streets of our city in those hectic final days before Christmas.

I learned.

All afternoon and into the early evening, we drove our way from lot to lot, examining tree after tree after tree. As the exasperated salespeople shook their heads in frustration, we explored every possible opportunity with no results. Nothing would match Poppy's idea of what her Christmas tree should look like.

"It's just not right," she said.

"Is there anything you like about it?" I asked.

"Well, it's straight. However, it's far too small. It would look so innocuous. It would get lost in my living room."

"Do you see one that's better?"

"No. This is ridiculous. Why don't they have a wider selection of trees? Why do they try to force people to buy trees that don't suit their homes?"

"Hmmm."

Eventually, as I teetered on the edge of physical and emotional exhaustion, we found a compromise. Better put, Poppy ran out of steam as well. It wasn't the perfect tree but it was an adequate tree. We looked at each other and shrugged. You can only talk so much about Christmas trees.

The tree salesman and I pushed it into the back of the station wagon. The next day Poppy and I started to decorate it. To Poppy, the decorating was extremely important. The tree had to look just so. She became the sorceress and I was the apprentice.

"Would you mind helping me fix the tree?" she said.

"Of course not, Poppy."

"You hold it."

I obeyed.

"To the left."

"How's that?"

"To the right."

"OK?"

"More to the left. You hold the lights."

I obeyed.

"Would you put that decoration there?"

"Poppy, could you tell me exactly where?"

"Right there. No, no. Over there."

Her finger zeroed in on one tiny branch, and to that branch, I moved.

Decorating the tree obviously thrilled her. I wasn't sure that she liked the tree all that much; nevertheless, she enjoyed bossing me around. It brought her great satisfaction. She was in control of the situation and ordering me about as if I were the underling. It was clear-cut: I am the controller – you are the controlled. No questions asked. I had seen enough of Poppy already to know that my role was not to contribute suggestions. She didn't want my ideas – she wanted my instant obedience.

I feared her reaction if I'd stepped out of line.

This is not to say she wasn't polite. Just the opposite. She knew how to manipulate people (in the best sense), usually without quite pushing them into the realm of rebellion. Her instructions were clear and concise, and if I had to question what she meant, there was no feeling of frustration in her reply. She patiently told me (or retold me) what she meant. Then we carried on.

We worked all afternoon on that tree. You might ask if we paused for a coffee break, as we worked away. No. Poppy never stopped. She was a woman possessed. It was non-stop until the tree was finished.

It was a sight to see. The finished tree was radiant – a miracle to behold. Easily one of the finest and most elaborately decorated Christmas trees I'd ever seen. When I left that evening, my heart was light. I was proud to be a part of raising that tree.

The next morning it was gone.

"Oh, what happened?" I asked, as casually as I could.

"Well, we just have to get a bigger tree. I felt that one wasn't big enough." The previous evening after I left, Poppy had decided the tree was not big enough and spent the night taking the decorations off and dragging the poor thing out in the back yard. She and Joanne from down the street had apparently argued over this decision. Joanne wanted to give it to someone who needed a tree. Poppy preferred to banish it to the garden. It was as if she wanted to punish it for being inadequate. Poppy prevailed, of course. The tree remained out there until well after the New Year. What a waste.

Meanwhile, off we went again to buy the biggest Christmas tree on the lot. We hauled it home, put it up, and trimmed it all over again. Indeed, it was the perfect tree. When you walked in that living room, you knew instantly that you were in the presence of one magnificent tree. Poppy was satisfied; indeed, very satisfied. There was no doubt it made her Christmas.

Shortly after the tree was in place, we went Christmas shopping. To put it mildly, this was a nightmare. We roamed up and down Yorkville Avenue and Hazelton Lanes checking out the shops. We were in and out of countless stores, and then we turned around and went back to the same places to look yet again. Poppy had no idea of what to give anybody. In most of the shops, we visited (and there were many), a clerk came over and offered to help us. Poppy was capable of being minimally polite: occasionally she responded that if she needed suggestions she would ask. More often, if a salesperson came over she said bluntly, "If I need your help, I will ask for it."

I have to say that Poppy wasn't normally rude to people… perhaps forward, but not overtly rude. She was well mannered and acted that way most of the time. She was the only person I ever met who could be rude to you with perfect manners. Arguably rude but technically not.

When she was pushing her cart in Summerhill Market, there was more than one instance when she came into conflict with someone else's cart in the narrow aisles. She was an 'I-was-here-first-so-get-out-of-my-way' type of person.

On more than a few occasions, she came dangerously close to making this a serious issue. Several times, I stopped and smiled to smooth things over. Thankfully, others were tolerant when we were not.

Returning to Christmas: When Poppy went shopping for cards, we entered almost every card store in the area and finally settled on something we'd looked at right at the beginning.

It was interesting to watch her because she knew she had to get cards and presents, but there was no real feeling behind her purchases. Was that simply Poppy's way, or was it the dementia taking its toll?

She performed the task; a chore that was completed properly was the only option. If not, then she wouldn't do it. She really didn't seem to care about the result. She was determined to do the chore correctly; she seemed oblivious of the delight her gifts might give her family.

When I started working for Poppy, the die was largely cast as to where she would go each day. She had a prescribed routine and she stuck to it religiously. As a result, it was easy for me to think that she really didn't have much of a problem. She might be overbearing and overly bossy, but that's hardly an illness. She handled routine decisions easily.

With the arrival of Christmas, however, we were into a realm of unfamiliar decisions. Christmas cards, the Christmas tree, and presents were new territory for her. She hadn't done those things in a year, while she shopped for groceries every day.

Therefore, I began to witness the side of Poppy that was under attack. Absent the familiar daily routine, Christmas was, in essence, new to her, and this is where her illness showed itself.

She had the same issues as anyone has at Christmas. What cards to get? What presents? You and I can figure this out relatively easily, though it may take a bit of thought. Poppy couldn't. She couldn't think it through. The once-a-year decisions of Christmas were inaccessible to her. It was evidently too much of a struggle to bring them back.

This must have been very frustrating for her. Poppy had lived through many Christmases and had likely seen herself as the leader in making the day a success. She had probably revelled in the sense of control it offered her.

Yet now she couldn't handle the decision-making role. On top of that, the growing sense of loss must have offered her intimations of a future day when even more of her life would disappear from her grip.

Fortunately, Anna called and told Poppy not to do any grocery shopping. She was coming for Christmas and would take care of that. That was fine with me; I was off for the period over Christmas and glad for a break from daily shopping.

On the twenty-second of December, I went down to Poppy's and met Anna for the first time. We had talked on the phone, but never in person. She was a beautiful, middle-aged woman, obviously very fit and healthy. We had a perfunctory hello and brief talk at the front door; Poppy did not even come to the door. I wished Anna a Merry Christmas and was off.

I found Anna's disinterest in me a bit peculiar at first, but realized that I was simply the latest of many of her mother's aides. In her mind, I might disappear as quickly as the rest. No matter. I was the helper and content to fill that role.

I don't think any of us, certainly not me, could have foreseen how involved I would become in this family's life over the next two years. No one could have predicted the rapport that would develop between Poppy and me.

That tree and its gorgeous trimmings? Poppy and I took it down after New Year's Day. The decorations had to be removed just so. Poppy loved the task, which took a whole morning. She enjoyed every minute. For her, it was like playing a game. There was no hurry and no sense of frustration. If the bulbs didn't fit in the box, she just kept trying until they did. She was a person who liked things (and people) in their proper places.

\*\*\*

# Emma

I had heard that a family friend was staying with Poppy several nights a week, so I wasn't surprised when one day, shortly before Christmas, Poppy and I arrived home from our afternoon shopping, and Emma was there to greet us.

"Robert, I presume," she said, and extended her hand. Poppy didn't say anything.

Emma is a tall, attractive woman. Her trademark is her long, gray hair, which she wears wrapped around her head in a manner that artfully sets off her dainty face. She always wears a loose- fitting, full-length skirt and flat shoes.

We chatted a little at that first meeting, and then I took off for home, little realizing how close our working relationship would soon become. Emma would prove to be one of the most caring and conscientious people I have ever known, and in addition, a marvellous partner in my efforts with Poppy.

Emma had lived in Rosedale most of her life but was now settled in the little town of Erin, just outside Toronto. Her mother currently lived in a Rosedale retirement residence, so Emma came to the city regularly to check on her.

Apparently, she had been looking around for a place to stay on those nights when it wasn't convenient to go home, and had reached an arrangement with Poppy through a family connection. She would stay with Poppy several times a month.

This proved to be an excellent plan. Poppy was fiercely opposed to anyone who even remotely resembled a caregiver or a nurse, so between daily visits from Laura, another long-time friend from across the street, and Emma's overnights, she was being observed without intruding on her sensitivities about needing help. Poppy always referred to Emma, and to anyone else staying with her, as 'guests.'

At first, Emma called me to check on what I was doing with Poppy on a particular day and when we were planning to be home. This gave her a chance to plan her own time, as there was no point in her hanging around the house alone if Poppy was not going to be there. As Emma and I got to know each other better, our contacts grew more frequent. She often gave me shopping suggestions. Even though Poppy controlled the shopping list, we often slipped things she'd forgotten into the shopping cart.

I soon realized that Emma knew Poppy better than anyone, was on the firing line on a regular basis, and seemed to be the one most responsible for Poppy. Therefore, a lot of my education about Poppy and her situation came from her. Emma gradually became the main coordinator of Poppy's day-to-day activities, with me to help execute the activities, drawn in as needed.

Though Poppy was adamant that she must set up all her own appointments, it was usually Emma (or I) who would actually book them.

Sometimes Poppy expressed indignation at an appointment she noticed in the book, and we reassured her that indeed, she had made that appointment and we had simply written it down for her.

"I don't remember that," she said.

"Yes, you made that appointment a few weeks ago."

"OK."

Poppy had a series of regular doctors' appointments, and we agreed that Emma should take her to these so that, as a woman, she could sit in on them in order to hear what transpired. Poppy of course was adamant that I must accompany them, so on doctor days, I claimed to be busy with something else and Emma would step in to fill the breach. That was acceptable to Poppy, and fortunately she never quite cottoned on to the fact that my mysterious other obligations always occurred on the days she was going to the doctor.

Part of Poppy's medical regimen involved regular visits to a psychiatrist. Emma told me once how the doctor had tested Poppy. He asked her to repeat all the words she knew beginning with the letter 'S.' Emma said she just about flipped because she knew (and feared) exactly what Poppy's first word might be. Poppy apparently paused, looked at Emma, smiled mischievously, and proceeded to rapidly list words beginning in S (omitting the big S word). The doctor finally had to interrupt to stop her. Emma said that the doctor stared at Poppy for an extra second and pursed his lips uncertainly. It was clear that he was surprised to find someone in her state so capable with words. This story left all of us scratching our heads about Poppy's condition.

Emma also was the main source of updates on Poppy's health for Jane, the social worker. Jane in turn would relay updates to Anna, in Utica.

After Jane moved to another position, Emma began contacting Anna directly and later on was in contact with her by telephone or email.

Meghan, who replaced Jane as the social worker, became the new link to the family. Anna had originally asked me to send her an email every week reporting on what Poppy and I did each day. I did that for about a month until we both agreed that it wasn't necessary. Poppy and I did the same thing virtually every day, so the repetitive emails were pretty well useless. From then on, I emailed Anna only when something special came up.

By April, Emma and I were working quite closely together. She had increased her stays to four nights a week, and was coming earlier and staying later in an effort to keep a closer eye on Poppy. She waited there in the morning until I arrived and then she went off on her own business.

Despite our close working relationship, I found that Emma and I had to be very careful interacting around Poppy. Poppy clearly preferred to feel that I was with her, not Emma. On a few occasions when I asked Emma a question, Poppy interrupted to say, "It really doesn't matter." As if to say, *ask me, not her.*

Poppy and Emma had a love/hate relationship. No matter what Emma said, Poppy said the opposite. They upset each other in equal proportions. Poppy could provoke Emma very easily, but God bless her, Emma would let it roll off her like water down the drain; then they forgot what they were fighting about and resumed their host and guest roles. I don't think many people could have put up with Poppy's behaviour as Emma did. Many of the caregivers quit for less.

Poppy and her meds were a constant source of friction. She had a blister pack for her pills and we regularly checked this out and queried her as to whether she had taken her medicine. Poppy reminded us that she was quite capable of taking her own pills.

"Well, are you sure you haven't already taken them?" Emma said.

"Of course I'm sure. Don't be stupid. I wouldn't take my pills twice."

"But today is Wednesday and it looks like you've already taken Thursday's pills. So what happened to Wednesday?"

Poppy shrugged. "So I got mixed up. So what?"

"But it doesn't help to take the meds twice."

"I don't need a lecture on this sort of thing."

Emma of course smiled sweetly through all this while Poppy fired up her famous glare. Their dancing around was something to watch. It was like two boxers sparring. Emma's perseverance on the issue was necessary. We often detected pill problems by Poppy's mood swings, or if Prince's behaviour seemed strange, then we knew that Poppy had accidentally dropped some pills on the floor. Sometimes it was like being on a roller coaster as Poppy became increasingly tense or more laid back and the dog's mood either matched hers or veered off in the opposite direction.

I often had to stop myself from laughing as Poppy and Emma interacted. They were very different personalities with different styles of doing things, yet they were in a circumstance where they really had to co-operate.

Sometimes things went awry. Emma is a friendly and outgoing person who loves to talk and interact with people. Long conversations are second nature to her. This drove Poppy nuts. Poppy was not interested in what she saw as idle chatter. She sat silent while Emma chattered away to me, glaring at Emma as if ready to leap across the table. It was funny. It was sad.

"How would you like to look at some horses, Poppy?" Emma said once.

"Why would I want to see horses?" Poppy retorted. "I grew up on a farm. I've seen enough horses."

I eventually developed a sense of when Poppy was getting 69
to the end of her patience with an interaction, and I backed
away. Emma was more determined. Emma, of course, was
just trying to be nice, and Poppy likely didn't really mean
to affront her. It's just that they had different styles. Emma
was sweet and pleasant and wanted to reach out to people.
She undoubtedly thought that talking and listening brought
people together in friendship. I often had a feeling that she
was making a deliberate effort to stimulate Poppy's brain
and delay the deterioration in her thinking. Poppy didn't
want stimulation, and if she had recognized that Emma
was trying to help her in this way, she would have had a fit.
Poppy wanted to get right to the point.

No nonsense. I often thought of that 'fifties TV detective
show, *Dragnet,* with Sergeant Friday who used to say, "Just
the facts, ma'am."

That was Poppy. Just the facts.

Hold the chatter.

Emma and I had a terrific relationship. She was very
giving. She called us Team Poppy. We had it down pat. We
could have taken on anyone. There wasn't a day we didn't
talk. Her greatest strength was her patience and tolerance.

One of Emma's secret weapons was her ability to look
sad. Emma could look sadder than anyone I ever met. When
she and Poppy had fallen into a monster argument, she
looked at Poppy with such a God-awful forlorn look on her
face. "Poppy, you shouldn't have done that," she whispered.

Emma's look of sorrow was very expressive. Sometimes she cried as well. Then Poppy realized she'd gone too far, and they hugged. At least Emma hugged. Poppy might throw her arms around her, but it was an embarrassed and perfunctory effort. Poppy was not the hugging type. In any case, it was an effort and showed that Poppy appreciated Emma's help. Then life continued as before. Poppy of course forgot the whole issue within minutes. Emma carried on as if nothing had happened.

I admired Emma's tolerance. I don't know if I could have been so forgiving if I had been in her shoes.

She was a saint.

***

# Life With Poppy

Working with Poppy and observing how she acted, I was learning first-hand how gradual the slide into Alzheimer's can be. It's like growing older. You don't notice it happening, but suddenly one day you look in the mirror and realize you've changed. Sometimes dramatically. It's the same with Alzheimer's, but the slide is far less manageable. With Poppy, it took me a long time before I could actually identify serious changes.

For example, when I first started with her, I didn't have a key to the house. That was understandable. I didn't need a key. Despite the diagnosis of Alzheimer's, Poppy seemed reasonably normal and was always there to let me in or out. After about three months, in early spring, she suddenly decided that I was to have a key. Motivation unknown. On the surface, she simply seemed to think it was more practical for me to let myself in when I arrived. It was part of a pattern of changes that suggested that the disease was tightening its grip.

Poppy kept her keys in the cabinet in the hallway. When we went out, she put them in her purse. Then she started leaving them in the buffet, and sometimes in her purse, and sometimes in the kitchen broom closet, and finally, all three, forgetting where she left them. For a short while, we resolved this problem by buying those colourful plastic stretchy key chains and attaching them to her purse.

Then keys started getting lost. Well, not exactly lost. Poppy lost a few keys, certainly. However, she began to give keys to the caregivers, and in addition, to the neighbours. I guess she thought that the key holders could race to her rescue if she ever got into trouble in the house.

In no time at all we went from a small number of keys in defined locations to a large number of keys scattered all over the place.

Poppy's zeal certainly compromised the security of her home. It seemed obvious that for safety and security, we should limit the number of keys available, and know exactly who had access to them. She had done the exact opposite. It seemed like everyone we knew had a key. Perhaps some we didn't know.

Poppy's locks were more sophisticated than the norm and required the owner to authorize duplication of the keys. Over time, the locksmith was making so many copies that, he insisted on calling Anna, Poppy's daughter, to verify that each duplication was permissible.

Another change: At first when we arrived home from our daily jaunts, Poppy jumped out of the car, gathered up her packages, and marched to her door unassisted. Over time, I began hauling her booty in, she unlocked the door, and I dropped everything in the vestibule. Later it evolved to where I helped her carry it all to the kitchen, and even later, started putting everything away. We never discussed these changes.

One day I arrived and an orange cat was waiting outside the door. I asked Poppy who she was and she said that it was Belle from next door. Poppy loved any animal, so Belle found the door open to her cries. She dashed in between Prince's legs with Prince in hot pursuit – not to fight, but to play. Apparently, Belle had been hanging around Poppy's house for quite a while and Prince and she were good friends.

Belle was a Burmese cat and extremely affectionate with everyone. Prince always perked up when Belle was around. I thought she had become Prince's best friend. However, Meredith, Belle's owner, was concerned. She often outside trying to find Belle. Eventually she realized that lucky Belle was spending most of her time inside with Poppy and Prince. Meredith certainly knew about and sympathized with Poppy's situation and her affection for animals. Nevertheless, she was upset that her own little cat was eating at Poppy's house, then going home, and turning up her nose at her own food. As well, there was also the frustration of never knowing where Belle was.

Meredith spoke to Poppy on several occasions, urging her not to let the cat visit. Poppy couldn't follow that kind of thinking. She loved the cat and enjoyed watching Belle play with Prince. Meredith never made this into a major issue, but it was a bit of a sore point.

Unfortunately, poor little Belle was killed crossing the street in front of the house. Poppy was very upset. She was morose for a few days. I asked the neighbours not to discuss it, but it became the talk of the neighbourhood and kept coming up again and again, prolonging Poppy's grief. The talk eventually petered out and Poppy forgot it. For once, her memory loss proved useful. This was the only time I saw her truly sad.

Poppy's short-term memory continued to falter. Emma drove a big SUV with a vanity license plate 1QT that stood for a religion to which she belonged. Seven times out of ten, when Emma pulled out of the driveway Poppy turned to me and said, "1QT – whatever does that mean?"

"Interesting."

Similarly, every time we drove down Jarvis Street, she questioned me about the huge, red, modern sculpture in front of a new condominium. I told her I didn't know any-thing about it, and that was it until the next time.

Gradually, Poppy began to relinquish some of her authority. First, she let me help determine the order of shops on our expeditions. This was a huge breakthrough. After that first delegation of authority, she let me plan new routes that took her to her favourite stores, but in less time.

Actually, after my going over her mail with her, the route plan was the biggest discussion we would have each day. Every morning I had to detail the plan to her before we set off. I had started as her helper and was now becoming her guide. Luckily, by this time Poppy seemed a lot more comfortable with most of my decisions. She was getting tired.

She still made her usual rounds: Summerhill Market, Ashbury Cleaners, Pet Valu, the shoemaker at Rosehill, Holt Renfrew, the hairdresser in Yorkville, and the Granite Club; this twice a week – once for a workout and once for badminton lessons. Drive, drive, drive. She was weary but relentless. Then she gave up fitness. She wouldn't admit it but I sensed that despite sharing some of the decision-making, she was simply finding it all a bit too much to deal with.

\*\*\*

# Summer Vacation Dreams

"Of course, I'll be driving to Maine for the summer."

About five months after I started, Poppy announced that she would be spending her summer, as usual, at her home in Maine. I'd seen pictures of this place around the house, and it was really something. Anna and Edward had told me how years ago Poppy's friend, Mary Johnston, had directed her to an historic, colonial-style house in southern Connecticut.

Poppy drove down to see it, fell in love with it, and subsequently had it taken apart stone by stone, board by board, and transported to northern Maine where she owned some oceanfront land. She had the house reconstructed and that was where she and her pets had spent virtually every summer since. That property was a major passion in her life.

I had no idea whether or not I would be going. Would she need me? Would I be staying in Maine for the summer?

I assumed that if she were going for the summer, someone would have to take care of her. I didn't question whether she was going or not. I had seen enough to know that what Poppy wanted, Poppy got. But not this time, or not quite, anyway. Anna got wind of the plan and there was a flurry of tense telephone conversations, which left Poppy in a very bad mood.

"Why can't I spend the summer down there?" she said. "I've done it many times before, I can do it again."

I didn't think she was really seeking my opinion, so I kept quiet.

"Sometimes my children don't understand me, that I like living alone, and have friends in Maine to help me."

Poppy was smoldering. I recognized that her attitude was: "Where there's a will, there's a way." She conjured up many arguments, but Anna, being from the same gene pool, countered them all. The telephone calls continued but Poppy's side didn't seem to be winning.

Finally, Anna came to Toronto. She and her brothers had discussed the situation and were convinced that it wasn't safe for Poppy to live in the Maine home all alone for a whole summer. As a compromise, Anna promised that Edward would arrange to spend the first three weeks of August there with her. Poppy, of course, found this unacceptable, and continued to argue vociferously for a more "normal" summer.

Whether Poppy agreed or not, the decision was made. Time sped by, we were suddenly into summer, and the issue more or less drifted away. Poppy grudgingly went along with it, but she was disappointed, and she felt the family was overreacting. I also felt that she realized her memory was not quite what it should be. She was starting to lean on me more and more. For example, if I made a suggestion now, she would not write it off out of hand. I think she also realized that she really had no choice. Something was better than nothing at all.

She had given in on a major issue. This was a rare occasion. Certainly since I had arrived, it was the first time. I think she felt overwhelmed. It was very hard to battle her children when they were so united.

As time went on and the disappointment faded, the idea that she would have Edward all to herself for three weeks really raised her spirits. She forgot about the lost summer and switched her focus to this grand vacation with Edward.

Meanwhile, Anna asked me if I would be willing to drive Poppy to Maine, and then return three weeks later to take her back to Toronto. I had always been on the periphery of these discussions.

Naturally, I agreed to take her. It seemed like a wonderful opportunity to see an area I'd never visited. It was a difficult assignment, given how Poppy could react to obstacles. It would also be a rigorous road trip, and she would be alone with me in the car for a prolonged period.

All my dealings on this issue were with Anna. Poppy and I never discussed the matter. Anna told her that I was driving her, and apparently, that was the end of it.

80     As the pets would take up much of the space in the back seat, we planned to use a Thule roof carrier to hold Poppy's clothes and personal things. The night before we were to leave, she and I got together to pack the Thule. We had a lot of trouble installing it onto the roof of the car, and had a series of discussions about this problem as we stood in the driveway. We both had a fair idea of how the roof carrier was supposed to be installed, yet neither of us could quite grasp the critical steps that were necessary to make it work.

As we tried to figure out which bar went where, she looked at me and said, "What do you think?"

This was a new Poppy. She had never been one for soliciting advice.

"I don't know, Poppy. Maybe this one goes over here."

"Try it," she said. "If it doesn't work, we could try that one over there."

She explained her point of view and I explained mine. We went back and forth for quite a while, sharing our ideas and trying to arrive at a solution. She listened to me and I listened to her. It was a real discussion.

"Poppy, are you sure that this key is the right one?"

"No. There could be another one. I'm not sure. Just try all the keys."

"That's a good idea."

"I'll go in the house and get the other keys."

She came back.

"You try them," she said.

Luckily, we eventually found the right key.

Poppy was delighted. I believe she was feeling that maybe
it was her fault that we didn't have the right key in the first
place. I also discovered that she could be a good team player
when necessary. This was a two-person job, and both of us
were really flying by the seats of our pants. We tossed ideas
back and forth. There was no control issue. It was a side of
her I'd never seen.

I also think that given Poppy's mindset, she was very
excited about this trip and realized that I was an essential
part to helping her get there. She knew that she needed to
work with me to make it happen. Therefore, she did.

If you had been there, you would never have dreamed
that there was anything wrong with this woman. Mentally
and physically, she was totally engaged and fully cognizant
of how to work with me to figure it all out. I was amazed,
frankly. Also exhilarated.

Our relationship seemed to grow enormously that
evening. From being her dutiful helper, I had been pro-
moted to a colleague. I felt good about myself and I felt good
about her.

Emotionally it was a strange place to be. My initial
naiveté was wearing off as I recognized that she did indeed
have memory problems, and that they were progressively
growing worse.

Balanced against this, I could see her isolated and com-
manding nature starting to soften as she realized she couldn't
carry on without help. I was a large part of that help. Instead
of being merely a 'go-fer,' I gradually found myself the one

person she could trust and get along with as she ventured deeper and deeper into this war with her mind. I felt like I was making a difference – a real contribution to her well-being. Moreover, she seemed to be aware of it. I looked forward to our road trip.

When I arrived the next morning, Emma was there to see us off, bringing sandwiches she had made for our lunch. We fiddled around for a while with the final packing and getting the dog and the cat into the car.

I felt like a million dollars as we drove down Highland Avenue in the gorgeous sunshine. It was fun. It was bizarre. I thought back to all the warnings I'd been given about Poppy and about all the staff who had quit, and I realized I was happy. It was like going on a trip with a friend. Far from fearing her wrath, I had now moved to the point where I quite enjoyed her company. She seemed at peace, having her dog and cat with her, as we headed to her Shangri-La in Maine and her wonderful son. She started digging out the maps and we set out along the Queen Elizabeth Way.

\*\*\*

# The Trip to Maine

There was a crippling line-up at the border at Lewiston. It was blazing hot and we must have sat there barely moving for a good hour and a half. Who knew what was going on? Nevertheless, the animals behaved perfectly – not a peep out of either of them. Poppy and I just relaxed, too. She said very little.

We watched a mini-soap opera as a driver with his family up ahead ran out of gas and pushed his car over the border. There was no way for them to get out of line, and there was no one they could turn to for help. We chuckled as the drama played out. I thought of turning on the radio at several points but held back. I don't like music in the car but I thought she might. However, she showed no inclination in that direction. We sat there and enjoyed our own thoughts.

84	Going through customs, I was edgy. You never knew when Poppy might say something that would bother people. The pleasure of the day prevailed, and she was polite and cooperative. She had an American and a Canadian passport. I told the border agent I was driving my friend to Maine. God knows what he was thinking about this senior couple heading down to Maine. Poppy was perfect. Anything to declare? Good as gold. It was a family scenario.

"Have a lobster in Maine for me," he said as he waved us on.

We took the state highway down to Anna's house in Utica, and Anna met us in her driveway. It was very hot so she was wearing a cool blouse and Bermuda shorts that showed off her muscular legs. She hugged her mother, then me. I was surprised. They didn't seem like a hugging type of family, but it was very kind of her.

Then Poppy gave me a big hug. This was very much unexpected. Poppy definitely was not a hugger. At least, not in my experience. What had I done to deserve all this affection? But why question good fortune and happy friends? Poppy and I seemed to be moving closer together, and that felt good to me.

"I hope you had an uneventful journey," Anna said.

I knew what she really meant and reassured her that all had gone well. Anna's two little children ran up to hug their grandmother, while Prince dashed around in circles, working off energy after his day in the car. We had a short chat in the driveway, but Poppy and I were both tired. I set out for my hotel, and Poppy settled in with her family.

I picked Poppy up early the next morning. Anna pulled me aside and told me she would leave shortly after us and get to the house to clean it up before we arrived. She wanted me to stall a little so she could get there a bit ahead of us.

We were off to the wilds of Maine. Back on the road again, Poppy assumed the role of navigator. She seemed like a good one, I must say. She was delighted to pore over the maps and direct our passage across the state.

Of course she loved being in charge. She tracked us from town to town. There are so many interstate highways in the U.S. which intersect each other so much that it's easy to get lost.

We drove past many towns that Poppy seemed to recognize.

"Poppy, how do you know all these places?"

"I know that town very well. I went to school there; boarding school."

At one point, she started singing. Something about, "Fifteen years on the Erie Canal, I had a great donkey and I had a great pal." I can't remember much of it but it seemed like some sort of folk song about the early days. It was amusing.

"Where did you learn that?" I asked.

"I don't know. I just know it."

I love driving and I love driving fast. The trick to driving fast is to fall in line with other speeders. Never be the one out in front to be picked off by the police. Better to be the follower who sails on by while the cop is preoccupied with the leader.

At one point, we passed a policeman by the side of the road and Poppy told me her story of getting stopped for speeding. She had been annoyed and asked the policeman why he had pulled her over. He'd said she was easy pickings, all alone on the highway, way over the speed limit. She had kept complaining and arguing, claiming that she had been confused because her Canadian car registered speed in kilometers per hour and the speed signs in the U.S. were in miles per hour. Apparently, the policeman got so frustrated with her protestations that he'd given up and let her go. Poppy was very proud of that success.

This was a rare occasion, for her to tell me a story about herself. It told me she was relaxed.

Later, we were up in the mountains and ran into some heavy rain. I came up behind a transport truck and swept out to pass it on a downhill stretch. However, I'd overlooked how fast these trucks accelerate when they're going downhill. As we came alongside the truck, the spray from the wheels enveloped us. I couldn't see much in front, or behind, or to the side. It was a dangerous situation and I wanted to get out of it as fast as possible. My experience has always been that when you are in a situation like that, you're damned if you do and damned if you don't. If the driver behind can't see you, then he's liable to rear-end you. The best thing is to step on it and get the hell away from it.

Which I did. 87

The Mercedes accelerated to more than 160 km an hour. In a few seconds, we were past and clear, but I waited anxiously to see if Poppy would comment, expecting her to complain about my speeding.

She didn't say a thing.

I glanced at her and she returned a mischievous smile. She hadn't moved a muscle. I'm a nervous passenger, though a confident driver. Poppy wasn't a nervous passenger at all. She liked the speed, I could tell. I think she missed driving. I almost asked her if she'd like to drive, but my better judgment prevailed and I didn't.

As we got farther up into Maine and started seeing signs for Bangor, the state capital, we both started getting edgy. The highway was going through increasingly desolate territory and there were fewer and fewer communities or even rest stops. It was a beautiful four-lane highway, but there was virtually no traffic.

Poppy pored over the map and I began to suspect she had lost track of where we were. She asked what the last turnoff had been. The fact was that we were getting closer and closer to Bangor, which is in the north, while her home was closer to Portsmouth, which is more southerly. The sun was starting to go down and we seemed to be in the middle of nowhere.

"We've come too far," she finally announced.

"We should stop and try to figure out where we are."

At the next turnoff, I pulled over. Poppy looked worried but I wasn't overly concerned. It was likely though that Anna would be anxious about us; she had only asked for a few hours' delay and we were giving her much more. I leaned over and peered at the map along with Poppy.

"Christ knows where we are," she said.

"Poppy, I think we need to talk to his father on this one."

She looked at me and laughed. "You're probably right," she said.

I'll never forget her laughter. She was so delighted to be lost and joking about it. I suppose she had confidence that I would somehow get us back on track.

A person always thrives on confidence.

"You know, my place is near Portsmouth," she said. "We've gone way past the turnoff."

"What is the turnoff?"

"I can't remember," she giggled. "But I'll know it when I see it."

This could have been a real mess, but somehow we turned it into another magical experience. Just as we had back in her driveway, installing the Thule, we worked together, discussing the alternatives, trying this and that, and gradually feeling our way along until finally we hit a highway that made sense.

I could tell that she was fully engaged in the exercise, and I certainly was too. It was yet another team effort.

"My home is down that way."

We approached the Highway One exit sign, and Poppy
recognized it as a road that would eventually pass by her
home. "If we can follow the old Highway One south around
the shore, then sooner or later we will come out at my house."

So, that's what we did. When I told people about this
later, they always assumed that I was upset over this screw
up. I suspect they were thinking I was a bit of a fool to let a
person with Alzheimer's take charge of the map reading.

Regret was the furthest thing from my mind. From my
point of view, Poppy had simply made an honest mistake.
We missed the turnoff. Northern Maine is like Northern
Ontario – not a lot of signs and a million trees that stretch in
every direction and look the same every mile of the way. No,
my mind always remains on the way we turned a problem
into a victory for both of us.

Back we came, and it only took us an extra three hours
to find her home. At one point, we took another wrong turn.
When you get into secondary roads in northern Maine, you
can get totally lost. Finally, we found a little town she knew —
from there she re-established her bearings, and we proceeded
to her place without further incident. It was just before a
little town called Demerascota. Pronounced "Demascota," as
Poppy insisted.

"We're very close now," she said.

We approached her home down a long lane. It was a
public road but there were only seven or eight homes in a
little community at the end. Poppy abruptly spoke up: "You
know my husband is buried over that hill."

"Oh."

End of conversation.

Poppy's summer place was a huge, two-storey home, authentic colonial cream with a dark-brown roof. There was a circular driveway, and a handsome barn off to the right. There were beautiful gardens – even when Poppy wasn't there she had people looking after them. The house was back a hundred feet or so from the ocean, and at high tide, the water would almost come up to it. Its grounds were very rocky, and it was a good-sized lot, maybe eight acres, landscaped to blend with the surroundings. It was very private. I could imagine that someone who craved solitude would really enjoy living there.

It was dark as we arrived. Anna came out the front door to greet us; our second encounter that day. As Anna approached the car, Poppy leaned towards me and suggested we not mention that we had gotten lost. I agreed. I knew that Anna would figure out the truth, but there was no need to highlight it.

Prince leapt out of the car and went crazy. We let Poppy's cat out and she raced into the house, up the stairs, and under a bed. Anna thanked me for the extra time.

"We got a little lost," I said.

"I figured that."

Then I was off to the nearby hotel, which they had arranged for me.

When I returned the next morning, Edward came out to say hello. He was a good-looking guy, early forties, my height, only slimmer and more muscular. I was impressed by how he treated his mother. He seemed to truly enjoy her. He hugged her and held her hand while we all talked. They seemed like a couple. He asked me how the trip had gone, and appeared genuinely concerned that his mother was all right and was being looked after. Poppy obviously returned the love.

Then I took off for Toronto.

When we said our goodbyes, Poppy hugged me again. "See you soon," she said.

I was very pleased with the journey. I felt that Poppy and I had gone beyond the driver/passenger relationship. I was flattered that we seemed to have become friends, and were a bit more of a partnership than we had been. Alzheimer's really didn't seem to be part of the equation. Our trip had been like travelling with anyone else you cared for. I knew this happiness couldn't last, that things were inevitably going to go downhill, but at that point, I was content to ignore that. There was so much pleasure in savouring the moment.

Driving home, I crossed over into Canada early and came through Gananoque and down Highway 401. I was glad everything had gone so uneventfully. Poppy had done very well.

Sure, we had gotten lost a few times, but I couldn't blame her for that at all. I supposed I should have done a better job of getting the directions in advance. Nevertheless, Poppy knew the way and if it hadn't been for missing that one turn, we would have been all right. The only thing that struck me as strange was that she had said so little. If I asked a question,

I got a short, polite answer. She rarely said anything she didn't have to. It occurred to me that perhaps she was really beginning to understand that there was something wrong with her, and she didn't want to expose herself to appearing foolish.

The next three weeks were a bit of a void. I missed seeing Poppy every day, and the shopping and adventures that went along with that. I was becoming part of her life, and I thought of her often. When I drove by one of our haunts, I would remember whatever had happened there. *That's Poppy. We went there.* It was like losing somebody even though I knew I was going to see her soon. Emma and I were in touch several times; she was housesitting Poppy's place.

Three weeks later, I drove down again to pick Poppy up. At the border, the guard looked at my papers and asked me what I was doing. "Is this your car?" he said.

"No, it belongs to the lady I'm picking up."

He was clever. He knew the car wasn't registered in my name. If I had been up to no good, he'd have expected me to claim it was mine. Fair enough.

I arrived at Poppy's house on another searing-hot day. The windows were open so they heard me and came out to greet me; Prince first, then Edward and Poppy. It was a bittersweet moment. They all looked very happy. Poppy seemed glad that I had come. She hugged me, and said it was nice to see me. All was well.

Poppy's long-time pal Mary Johnston was there also. I had a nice talk with her while Edward and Poppy were

getting things out of the house. For some reason, the topic of 93
Poppy's driving came up.

"Have you ever driven with Poppy?" I asked.

"Once," Mary said, and smiled. "And never again. I don't like to talk about it."

As Poppy and I drove back out to the highway, I remembered her earlier comment from when we drove in and said, "Would you like to visit your husband's grave?"

"No," she said.

She seemed content to be going back to Toronto. Edward had told me she'd spent a lot of her time at the local harbour talking with the fishermen and buying fresh fish for dinner.

I didn't dare to ask her if she'd had a good time. She would have simply said, 'Of course.' You didn't ask Poppy the obvious. She wasn't interested in the obvious.

Coming into Utica to see Anna we got lost again; we missed a turn. It was as much my fault as Poppy's, but she didn't care. We finally had to phone Anna for help.

"Anna, will you talk to your mother and sort out how to get to your place? She's the navigator," I said. Anna laughed and told us what to do.

Luckily, she didn't know that earlier in the day we had stopped to let Prince out of the car and discovered we had forgotten his leash back at the house. In desperation, I had pulled off my belt and used it as a leash each time we stopped on the rest of the way home.

Unfortunately, my pants were loose so without a belt I was walking around with my pants askew, holding them up with one hand and holding on to the belt with the other. It was very awkward, and we must have looked a sight to anyone passing by. Poppy did not have a belt herself and the dog needed its regular pit stops. We couldn't just let him run around on the highway.

Poppy was very grateful for my little sacrifice of dignity. She laughed at my predicament, and thanked me over and over. That was a rarity.

The trip home was Poppy at her best. Animals were supremely important to her. In her mind, I was helping her dog, and anyone who could help an animal was worthy of great respect. When we got home, we found the leash under some baggage. It didn't matter. It had all been good fun.

I phoned ahead to Emma when we got close to home, and she was out on the lawn waiting for us when we arrived. She gave us both a big hug. I helped Poppy collect her bags and carried them up to the door. Emma would take over from there. Laura from next door came over, to welcome us home. Poppy seemed relieved to be back in her familiar surroundings. As I turned to head off, she turned to me and smiled. "Now that we're here why don't you come in and have a drink?" she suggested.

I was flabbergasted. She had never offered me a drink before.

"Poppy, I'd love to, but I'm driving and really tired. Let me call you tomorrow morning."

Despite my refusal, I was thrilled. Obviously, Poppy was seeing me in a new light. All sorts of people commented in the weeks that followed, that something had happened on the trip that won Poppy over. Meghan, the social worker, told me she was amazed to have Poppy rave about me to her, where previously I had been more or less just part of the scenery. Emma made the same sort of comment, and so did Laura.

"What did you do on that trip?" Meghan asked.

"I don't know. Nothing special."

Thinking about it later, I felt that Poppy appreciated the relaxing time, and associated it with me. I suspect that most people with Alzheimer's don't have much time to relax. There are always pills to take, chores to do, questions to ask, and appointments to attend. I didn't create any problems for her. We talked occasionally when needed, but generally, she sat there and let her mind roam. I became one of the few people with whom she could be at ease. She felt comfortable with me.

I went from being an assistant to being a friend. From then on, I could do no wrong. Naturally, this would upset the other caregivers. But that's another story.

That trip was also a tipping point. From then on, Poppy became a lot more dependent on me. I was never sure whether she trusted me more, or if it was simply a case of needing me more. Once a very independent spirit, she was suddenly willing to lean on me much more often.

I also had a feeling that she was happy to be back in Toronto because she felt safer there. Maine was a little too close to Hartford, and Hartford, she knew, was where her

96     children would most likely put her in a nursing home. In Toronto, she was in a stronger position to fight this battle.

For the moment.

# Life Becomes More Difficult

In the beginning Poppy had known exactly what she wanted and would tell me what I had to do to make it happen. This changed into her telling me what to do, and if she couldn't remember exactly what that was, she would let me fill it in and would carry on as if there was no gap at all. Now she seemed willing to leave many more decisions to me.

At the same time, our shopping trips became more and more selective. They narrowed down to a precious few places – the Summerhill Market, the pet store for cat food, the vet's office for dog food, the fish market on Bayview, Starbucks for her coffee, and the drycleaners. She had let old haunts slip away, I suspect, reflecting her diminishing interest in her surroundings.

Soon after we returned from Maine, she began to have problems with her contact lenses. She was losing them all the time, leaving them in overnight, or inserting them inside out. When I discovered these problems, we went to her regular optometrist, who checked her out and ordered up new packages of contacts. Of course she lost them and had to go back and buy some more. This happened several times.

The optometrist decided it was bad for Poppy's eyes to be misusing the contacts this way, so she started leading Poppy towards wearing glasses. I knew Poppy was still rather vain about her appearance, and would not take kindly to this suggestion. I mentioned this to the technician, and asked if there was a way she could introduce the notion as delicately as possible. The technician looked at me as if I were trying to take over her job, and charged ahead. Of course, when they started trying on glasses, Poppy became belligerent. For some reason the technician could not bring herself to explain what they were doing and why. She just wanted to get glasses on the old lady. Well, that old lady saw no reason to switch from contacts.

"I not only know what I want but I know what I don't want," Poppy said, scorching her with that glare. The technician cringed and became speechless. I went over and suggested we leave. Poppy stood up and stormed out. She was furious. On the street, she announced that she would never go there again. "I don't need glasses anyway," she said.

Her eye problems continued, however, and a few days later, I proposed a place that I liked – Yonge Vision on Yonge Street at Davisville. That owner had a completely different

attitude. I mentioned Poppy's sensitivities, and he assured
me that he dealt with people like her on a regular basis.

Poppy had a slight eye infection due to wearing the same
contacts too long, so this gentleman advised her to try wearing
glasses for just three or four days while the inflammation
cleared up. This elementary logic (and, I suspect, the fact that
he was a man) made all the difference in the world to Poppy.
She took the glasses, wore them for the prescribed time, got
used to them and never mentioned a desire for contacts again.

When we ordered the glasses, I suggested, based on our
previous experience with keys, watches, and sunglasses, that
she should buy three pairs with identical frames so there
would be no confusion. If we lost a pair, we would use one
of the spares and buy time until we could locate the missing
one. Now we could say, "I found your glasses," and she
would accept that. We couldn't lose them all at once. Well, I
suppose we could, but I kept one pair in the car so at least I
knew where that one was.

At the pet store, I always waited at the front of the store
while she went to the back to select cat food. I was never,
even at the worst of times, allowed to go and help select the
food myself or even witness the deliberations. She didn't
need my help. I didn't know her cat as she did. When we
got to the cash register, she often faltered: "I can't find my
credit card."

"Try looking in your wallet in your purse – that's where
I would look."

Yes, that's where it was.

Emma, who had originally been staying over a couple of times a week, gradually increased her time until it turned into five nights a week. Anna and her brothers realized that Emma couldn't be present all the time, so they hired professional caregivers to come in two or three nights a week. Then they saw that Poppy needed even more care. Soon we had fulltime caregivers.

Unfortunately, the caregivers usually couldn't take it for more than a few days. They did the best they could, but Poppy simply couldn't abide their presence or anything they tried to do for her. They complained that there was no rest while dealing with her and that nothing they did was acceptable. She was always getting mad at them. Poppy got frustrated with the way they did things, or failed do them. One time, one of the caregivers complained to me about how she had gone downstairs to get a second cup of coffee and Poppy had said, "Don't touch that – it's for him."

'Him' was me.

The caregivers were right. Virtually everything they did annoyed her. They would look at me and shrug in frustration. I didn't know what to do. I kept quiet. I didn't agree with Poppy, but to me there was no point in antagonizing her.

She was adamant that she must answer the door herself. On the odd occasion when the caregiver got to the door ahead of her, she bluntly reminded her not to do that. Poppy didn't like being looked after. She clearly would have been happier being on her own. Her attitude seemed to be,

'This is my house, and these people are visiting me, and it's none of their business what I do.'

She didn't like me associating with the caregivers. In later months, Poppy became more and more suspicious, saying, "What are you two talking about?" when we had our little meetings. She resented the caregivers more and more, and she became friendlier to me.

Laura, her next-door neighbour, was a true, dear friend, and she dropped in to check on Poppy almost every day. Laura often suggested things for Poppy to do. For example, she might bring some books for her to read. Poppy loved reading, but only her own choice of book. She argued with Laura over why she should read Laura's recommendations. Poppy shot down Laura's critique, explaining why she wouldn't read a book like that. They often ended up in an argument that turned into a shouting match, which, funny enough, they both seemed to enjoy thoroughly.

One day I went to make coffee, which to Poppy's mind was her job alone. She knew how the machine worked. I didn't. She yelled at me and the glare came out. I shared my own glare with her. I thought I was doing her a favour, but obviously she disagreed. Thankfully, she seemed to instantly recognize she'd gone too far. "I can talk to you that way," she said. "You're just one of the family."

I chose to take that as a compliment, and she never yelled at me again.

Her charity-giving gradually turned into a significant problem. She had always spent a lot of time in her office writing cheques to the various animal charities that had learned of her susceptibility to their message. Many of these organizations wrote to her to express their thanks, and Poppy unfortunately responded with yet another cheque. Her daughter Anna eventually noticed this from the bank statements and put a hold on that kind of enterprise.

Then a more serious problem arose – Poppy began to forget her appointments. Originally, she kept a very strict day-timer, but as time went on, she often wrote her appointments in on the wrong day or time. Gradually Emma and I had to take charge of her calendar, though Poppy never willingly relinquished that responsibility. We always had to do this surreptitiously, which was quite a game. She was perpetually amazed at how we knew what she was doing, and we assured her that she had made every appointment herself.

Even as we struggled to keep track of her appointments, Poppy increasingly decided at the last moment not to attend whatever was on the calendar. This included not only the medical appointments but also the social dates. I am told that this is typical of Alzheimer's: Your friends sense that you are no longer there when they're with you, so they stop calling. When they stop calling, then you lose what little interest you had in their presence. This is the maddening part. When I first met Emma, she told me that Poppy's social life had already dropped by about seventy percent. Now it was even worse.

I don't think Poppy ever acknowledged she had any troubles. She liked to think that she made her own decisions, and that's what she was doing. On the other hand, perhaps she was feeling embarrassed. The more I think about it, it was clear that something was wrong but it wasn't out in the open. When you're living in something, you sometimes don't think about it.

I can see now that she was always tense. Was this her personality or was she nervous that others would see there was something wrong? After a life as a leader, it must have been painful to let people witness her confusion.

She loved structure. She was quite happy doing the same round of stores every single day and buying the same things at every shop. If I didn't call by 9:30 a.m., she would be on the line to me in minutes.

She seemed determined to keep her routines intact. To diverge was to lose ground. It wasn't totally downhill though; shortly after we returned from Maine, I invited Emma and Poppy for dinner at my daughter's home where I was house-sitting. The house had three cats and a dog, so Poppy was in her element. The dog was a cross between a Malamute and a Husky; a magnificent animal. Poppy was so happy and so gracious that one would never have suspected there was anything wrong with her.

Later on in November, Emma, Venitia (the only caregiver she ever found acceptable), and I organized an American Thanksgiving dinner. For once, Poppy just sat back and let us do everything. She was queen for an evening. We cooked up a wonderful turkey dinner with all the trimmings.

As she slipped deeper into dementia, Poppy increasingly trusted and relied on me. We seemed to know each other better. I sensed that I gave her a feeling of safety, that she knew there was someone who cared and watched out for her.

The unpredictability of life with Poppy created a sense of excitement, confusion, and challenge. While I am sure it would not have struck Poppy this way, Emma and I never knew what she would be up to next, but it was almost guaranteed that something would emerge and we would find ourselves rallying for yet another attempt to save the day. It was sad, but it was fun.

Strange . . .

\*\*\*

# The Cat

Poppy had a cat named Samantha. She was an overfed and unsociable beast, which lived in Poppy's bedroom. During the day, she slept on a chair by the window and rarely came out of the room. Keep in mind, Prince was always there wanting to play if the cat came out, and this cat didn't want to play.

Samantha was a very serious Siamese. If you came upon her accidentally, she just looked at you and walked away. I give her credit for not biting, but otherwise she wanted nothing to do with people. I never felt the need to pat her and I doubt if she regretted my reticence.

Poppy adored Samantha. This was her cat. No one else was to care for her. No one else was to feed her. No one else was to change the litter. The cat was sacrosanct, and woe betide the hapless individual who tried to assist or intervene in the care of this feline devil. This was the rule, from the first day I worked with Poppy, to the last day of our time together.

You were flirting with real and present danger by going anywhere near that cat. Occasionally, one of the new caregivers who liked cats set out to clean the litter box. That would only happen once because Poppy let her know to keep her hands off. There were rules. It was her home and she was the boss.

Early on in my sojourn, I had the temerity to suggest that I could pick up the cat food for her. Poppy froze me in her icy glare and said, "I know more about Samantha than you, and I know what she likes and doesn't like."

Silence – end of that lesson.

Our twice-weekly visit to the pet store to buy cat food was a highlight for Poppy. She always left me in the car (or later, at the front of the store), and headed off to the back where she could pick over the tins for twenty or thirty minutes until she had pulled together a collection that she was convinced the cat would like.

Unfortunately, despite her confidence about understanding the cat's needs, I eventually recognized that Poppy had never truly figured out what the cat really wanted. The cat nibbled at this and nibbled at that, and if she didn't like how it tasted, that food was destined for the garbage. Then off we went to the pet store to buy more. It was a circus.

It never changed. We bought a dozen or so cans of food, twice a week, and just as regularly, threw it away.

A tremendous amount of money was shooting out the door. I told the people at the pet store that logic had nothing to do with this. Just don't say anything, I told them, and they took that advice to heart. They went out of their way to accommodate her. I must say that this was just about the only area of Poppy's behaviour that I found ridiculous. It was understandable, given her illness, but still ridiculous.

Was this the original Poppy or Poppy altered by disease? I'd like to blame it on the disease. How could the woman who I found so interesting and vital fall prey to such foolishness? In truth, in talking with the others, the message seemed to be that Poppy had always been this way with the cat. So be it. Everyone is entitled to an idiosyncrasy or two, I suppose. This was Poppy in spades.

\*\*\*

# Shopping

Her shopping list represented one of the most reliable barometers for tracking Poppy's slow decline. She insisted on shopping for fresh food every day. Frozen or canned was unacceptable – it had to be fresh. So one of our principal stops was the Summerhill Market, a mid-size, upscale gourmet food store cum supermarket in the north end of Rosedale. Read: High End. Expensive. Cost didn't matter to Poppy. It was in stores like this, and a few others, that some of our most poignant adventures played out.

As I've said, in the beginning Poppy maintained exclusive control of the shopping list. She had it already prepared when I arrived in the morning, and she knew exactly what she wanted. When we got to the market, she went in while I waited patiently until she emerged with bags and bags of groceries.

Later on though, I recognized that things were not working out quite right. One day, I took my own little shopping list from home and went into the market after she had gone in. When we met in the aisle, she was suspicious, but when I explained I was just doing my own shopping she nodded. That went on for about a month until we drifted into my going in with her and walking around with her. I was strictly looking after my own shopping, of course, so she didn't feel she was being watched. That seemed to satisfy her. In fact, I had a growing sense that she was glad to have me there. She just didn't want to admit it.

The shopping gradually occasioned more discussion. I noticed that she was not only buying everything on her list, she was also buying more and more things that she just spotted in the store. She started asking me what I thought of this and what I thought of that. She was bored with the same old veggies, she would say, and I would suggest something new. Occasionally, she agreed.

She liked to use only the plastic hand baskets provided, and she could get away with that, as she was very strong. I pushed a cart. Finally, one day, I said, "Poppy, do we really need the basket? The cart might be easier."

She put the basket back in its place and from then on, I pushed the shopping cart and she collected the food and filled up the cart. Eventually I took over the list and we both studied it and collected what she needed.

As time wore on, she became increasingly sensitive to very small matters.

Buying some cobs of corn turned into a long discussion
about why they always packaged the corn cobs in threes.
Poppy was certain that shoppers wanted two or four cobs
– they didn't want three. She insisted that it was idiotic to
force people to buy three.

One time she went to the head of the vegetable department and argued quite forcefully that she wanted only two
cobs – one for herself and one for her guest. He looked at
me somewhat askance; I shrugged, and he went away and
returned with a package of two he had made up especially
for her (she was a much appreciated customer). From then
on, every time we went we had this same discussion and she
insisted on having two especially packaged for her. To me,
this endless, repetitive debate seemed to be a bad sign.

There was another day when she opened up a package
of raspberries, tasted a couple, pronounced that they weren't
quite ripe, and put the package back in its place.

She drove the fellow at the fish counter crazy. Being from
Maine, she was accustomed to fresh seafood and knew a
great deal about it. She asked the poor fellow detailed questions about the seafood, and he often had no idea what the
answer was. She wanted to know the difference between different kinds of salmon. She wanted to know what area the
clams came from. When he told her one type of oyster was
sweeter, she insisted on tasting both oysters and had to agree
with him. She knew her fish and other seafood.

At the Summerhill Market, she questioned the cheese
server in the same way – something about the difference

between French and German blue cheeses. Which was stronger? The woman clearly didn't know, but Poppy was an excellent customer and so intimidating, that the lady opened up both packages, laid a slice of each on a plate and invited her to decide for herself. Issue resolved.

We moved on to the evening's dinner. "Who's eating with me tonight?" she asked. "Why are they with me?" This would lead into an interminable debate. "How do you know they like this?"

"They told me. You had it last week and they liked it," I said.

The same question about her "guest" came up virtually every day. Curiously, some days she seemed concerned, and other days she didn't seem to worry at all. "I don't like that and I don't care," she said.

Even today, I could go in and shop for Poppy. Despite all the time we spent on the list, it never really varied much: mushrooms, fish and meat, veggies, strudel, Chelsea buns, jam and butter tarts.

One evening I got home and Stephanie pretended to bow to me. "How is my little gourmet shopper tonight?" she said.

"Oh brother, give me a ham and cheese sandwich any day. Something simple."

***

# Food

Poppy loved to eat. You wouldn't know it to see her – she was so slim and fit. Food was one of her main interests. Unfortunately, she was also a tad demanding in what she ate and how it was procured and prepared.

Remember that she was a wealthy woman and had long been used to fine foods and service. She had developed standards over the years, and she definitely wasn't going to relinquish them. Money for groceries meant nothing to Poppy. She rarely noticed cost. If she wanted it, she bought it.

She spent an enormous amount on food each month and simply put it on the credit card. Her grocery bill was quite astounding, but Anna took care of all her Visa charges so that Poppy never really saw the result of her spending.

I remember one time, and it was the only time, that she was hung up on the cost of something. She picked up some strawberries and said they cost too much. She put them back and that was it. It never happened again.

Poppy's breakfast was always three or four thick slices of toasted French bread with a slab of butter on each, topped with a dollop of jam; strawberry, raspberry, or blueberry, with a large cup of coffee or two. She loved her coffee. She took it very strong, but laced with cream and sugar. She ground this coffee herself.

While eating breakfast she read the *Globe and Mail* cover to cover. Every so often, she said,

"What do you think of that?"

This wasn't a signal that she wanted to talk about whatever world event had captured her attention. Quite the opposite. The truth was she usually forgot what she had read almost instantly. She read the paper, and then read it again. She forgot it all. I responded to these invitations with the shortest of answers. "Yes, interesting." That was all she needed or wanted. Any more would expose her problem. I thought she was really saying, 'I want to discuss this, but I can't.'

Lunch at home was often a slice of smoked salmon (at fifty dollars a pound) plus a couple of bits of Chelsea bun, a butter tart, and a glass of white wine. She usually ate standing in the kitchen – lunch for her was merely something you had to have as a mid-day snack.

In the early days, Emma occasionally took her to a coffee shop over on Broadview, where many of Emma's friends liked to gather to talk. Poppy enjoyed getting out and mingling with these people, but she would never stay for lunch. If pressed, she would say, "No, I don't eat lunch."

Home she went, to grab her 'snack' standing up in the kitchen.

Lunch wasn't important; breakfast and dinner were her serious meals. Emma used to tell me about their dinners. It was always a regal meal with fish or meat or fowl. If meat, the steaks had to be rare. Poppy wanted her steak cooked maybe fifteen seconds a side and that was fine. She thought you ruined meat by cooking it very much. Properly cooked meat for her meant blood red.

Poppy loved bread. She always had to have Chelsea buns, strudel, croissants, and French baguettes. They weren't very healthy, but they were her staples. Oh, and butter tarts, I nearly forgot. She could never be without butter tarts.

Every day we bought two French sticks. (We didn't need them and would often not use them.)

"Poppy, do you really need two of them?"

"Well, just in case."

"I think we have some in the freezer already."

"Are you sure?"

"Yes, I'm sure."

"Well they probably aren't fresh so we'll get a couple just in case."

We ended up throwing out at least half of the French bread we bought. If I suggested butter tarts, then she said, "I don't need butter tarts every day." We bought them just in case.

Every so often, she seized on the notion of cooking up some complicated recipe that she had found in one of her cookbooks, and insisted that we gather all the ingredients at the market. I didn't say much, but I knew the caregiver did not want to tackle such a difficult task. That didn't matter. The caregiver simply fashioned the ingredients into something plain and simple under Poppy's watchful eye, and Poppy accepted that without dispute.

She drank only white wine, but she had red for her 'guests.' She ended up with quite a stockpile of red, as we always had to buy a bottle or two when at the liquor store; even though I told her she had plenty. She always wanted to be sure. Some of her guests did drink red, so there was some justification for her purchases.

She was possessive of her kitchen. We shopped and then put all the food away. No one was allowed to touch anything. She insisted on washing the dishes, or at least on running the dishwasher.

Caregivers were prohibited from using the dishwasher. She didn't even let them in the kitchen while she was cleaning up. She told them to get out.

Much later, she let them make dinner and clean up, but she stood there watching and providing a running critique of what they were doing.

As time went on, she became more and more erratic in the kitchen. She took something out of the freezer, thawed it, then refused to eat it, and put it back in the freezer. Once she bought some expensive smoked salmon, and left it in the fridge for days. Then she opened it up, tasted it, didn't like it, and asked me to taste it to see if it was still all right.

I said, "Poppy, there's no point in both of us getting sick if it's not OK."

She looked at me thoughtfully and nodded her agreement. "Hmmm, good idea. That makes sense."

She ate it, with no dire consequences, I might add. She had a cast-iron stomach. We were all afraid to put our hands in the back of the fridge. You never knew what kind of mouldy mass you would find.

\*\*\*

# The Second Christmas

I was not looking forward to our second Christmas season together. The first had really been an ordeal, what with the endless shopping for Christmas cards, presents, and the famous Christmas tree. I could only envisage our second Christmas as even worse. To my surprise, the interest *or lack thereof* came from an entirely new direction.

"We really must start getting ready for Christmas," she said every few days.

"Yes, I agree."

Nothing happened.

Her behaviour was quite different that second Christmas. Whereas the previous year she had been consumed by the drive to fulfill all the obligations she identified with Christmas, the second year she seemed to have only a vague notion that she should do something, but she wasn't quite sure what that was. Better put, she knew she needed to do certain things for Christmas, but she seemed to lack the mental energy to get down to it. As time passed, it became evident that she wasn't willing to put an effort into any of the previous year's pursuits.

She left it too late to buy Christmas cards and we never even discussed a tree. The only presents we bought were for Anna's son and daughter. Anna had prompted Poppy as to what the kids might like – specific books from Mabel's Fable's – and we ended up driving to their store on Mount Pleasant where the kids were registered. That was it. Nothing else.

She did ask me how much to tip the caregivers. I wrote them each a Christmas card of thanks and put in a hundred dollars. I really didn't know what to give them. It's tough when you're dealing with someone else's money. You don't want to throw it around, but you don't want to appear cheap.

There was another reason for Poppy's lack of interest in pre-Christmas chores. Edward was coming to stay with her for Christmas, and Poppy was focused on this stay. She talked about his visit every day, and nagged the caregivers incessantly to make sure that his bedroom was properly made up. She was eagerly looking forward to going out to dinner with him and seeing some theatre.

Christmas was way out of Poppy's comfort zone. Even at its best, Christmas can be a trying and exhausting experience. I suspect that for her it was pleasant to let the trials of Christmas just slip away, and to relax in her precious time with Edward.

You might ask what being 'excited' might mean for a person like Poppy who was so controlling of her own emotions. I would have to say that excited for her would be much like you or I acting normally. It wasn't a highly visible display of emotion. She didn't wave her hands, cheer, or do any of the traditional things most of us do to convey our extreme engagement. You could tell very little from her voice. It was more the sense of urgency she brought to the task. She became very detail-oriented. Everything had to be just so.

Everything had to be perfect for Edward. Every meal had to be planned in advance. Just in case. Make sure we have enough…of everything.

I confess I felt the enthusiasm in her presence, rather than in her actions. I had spent so much time with her that I could sense her feelings even when most others could not detect anything out of the ordinary. This might, of course, mean I was misinterpreting her.

However, I don't think so.

We had to have new bed linens for Edward, and so we spent nine hundred dollars on bedding. The packages almost filled the back of the car. Anna got a shock when she saw the credit card bill and phoned to ask me about it. As far as she was concerned, her mother's house was full of usable bedding. I explained that I had taken Poppy out, but couldn't stop her buying. Anna was upset, but said she realized it wasn't my fault.

In her anticipation of Edward's visit, Poppy thought carefully about what he might like to eat.

Really, it was as if we were shopping for a huge family. She wanted to cover all the bases, so the obvious solution was to buy everything. She never seemed to think of calling Edward and asking him what he wanted. It was easier just to buy it all.

I guess I sound a bit dismayed about the way we shopped for the Christmas food, but in truth, it was a lot more exciting than our usual routine and I welcomed that. After all, we were still trooping off to Summerhill every day and going through the same numbing rituals around the fruit and vegetables.

"Should we get some apples?"

"Maybe," I'd say. "What do you think?"

"Perhaps. What about some peaches?"

"You like peaches."

"Oh no, they don't look good at all."

"Would you like some cherries?"

"No. No cherries. I've never liked cherries."

"So what would you prefer?"

"What about some pears? Would my guests like some pears?"

We went on and on debating over every fruit in the store (and even some they didn't have), and in the end she bought what she always bought. Then she turned to the vegetable aisles and went through the same routine.

I was off over Christmas, so I can't report on much that happened, except for one shocking incident. A few days after

Christmas, I arrived at the door (Edward had already flown home) to be greeted by Poppy wearing dark glasses.

"Nice to see you," I said. "Hope you had a good time over Christmas?"

"We had a wonderful time," she said. Then she took off her glasses.

"My God, Poppy, what happened?"

"I fell."

"It must have been quite a fall."

I wasn't exaggerating. She was a mess. She had two terrible black eyes and scratches all over her face. She looked like she had been in a bar-room brawl.

It was awful.

"I tripped on the steps just outside the front door," she said.

"I hope you haven't broken anything."

"No, no. I didn't want to go to the doctor but they made me. I'm fine. It doesn't look very nice but I'm OK."

Well, that was an understatement. She looked like a raccoon.

It turned out that Poppy and Edward had gone to a family friend's cocktail party. On the way out, Poppy had fallen flat on her face on the steps. Fortunately, she wasn't hurt badly and she looked far worse than she really was. She was glad it had happened at the end of the holiday rather than at the beginning, so fewer people would see her.

This fall may not have been serious physically, but it really seemed to affect her confidence. Her attitude changed.

124    She was not as sure of herself in many ways. She was more withdrawn. Something more than physical pain had happened there, and it was more than vanity too. Every time she looked in the mirror, she was looking at a woman in serious trouble — a woman in fear of her family using this as an excuse to spirit her away from her home.

For the first few weeks after that, she wore the dark glasses when we went shopping. The problem, however, was that when she had to read something in the store, she had to remove the glasses, and anyone at hand immediately noticed her bruises. This became a real annoyance to her.

You might wonder how someone with Alzheimer's would fare at a sophisticated cocktail party. I was told she had a gratifying time. She was always a bit of a party girl, of course, and she was very adept socially. She could still turn it on when required. She could meet you and you wouldn't know anything was wrong.

Sometime after Christmas, I had a friend come in to help fix her antique clock and Poppy was charming. The two of them had a good time, and I am sure he was wondering how this woman could have Alzheimer's and still function so well. When he asked her about the clock, though, the truth became a little more evident. She couldn't remember any of the clock's history — where she had bought it, how old it was, what style it was. That's where the Alzheimer's showed. She could be perfect socially, acting interested and gracious, yet couldn't remember details. Nor did she seem to care. It was incidental to her. It didn't cross her mind that

she should remember this. You or I might have remembered    125
at least a few details of something like an antique clock. She
unfortunately remembered nothing.

They say that with Alzheimer's, until it is really advanced
you have some long-term memory, but a very weak short-
term memory. However, if something is repeated often
enough, it moves from short-term memory to long-term
memory. I saw this often with her. I imagine that's why
Poppy liked to do the same things every day. Anything new
was outside her comfort zone.

\*\*\*

# Later Days

Poppy's problems accelerated dramatically in the spring of 2011. In the early days, she had decided on every item on the grocery list. Gradually, that had turned into a form of collaboration with each of us contributing to the list equally, and then it slipped further to where I was making seventy-five percent of the decisions. Finally, we reached the point where I simply wrote out the list, and she watched. It was so much easier for both of us.

She sometimes went to the fridge to check on my list, and was surprised that I was right about what was needed. At this point, I was deciding on almost everything, and she seemed content to go along with that. I still treaded very softly. I would never just come right out and say, 'Bang, bang, bang – this is what we need.'

That would have only brought on an angry response: "Don't tell me what I need."

Instead, I always put it to her in terms of a question or a suggestion. Then she could nod her head in agreement. Sometimes, if she was a bit doubtful about my recommendation, I might soften it a bit by saying, "I'll just put it down for now. We may not need a Chelsea bun but we can decide later."

She agreed to that most of the time...but not always. Her mood really altered when we talked about supper. We had a major discussion on who would be there, what was best for them, how much we needed. And so on. Of course, there were only ever two people, and such a discussion was rather over the top. Nevertheless, she seemed to need it.

Sometimes she was very concerned about what her 'guests' (Emma or the caregiver) would want to eat for supper, while at other times she would get very irritable. "I don't care what they want – I'll make the decisions about what they eat."

Sometimes she tossed the decision to me; other times not. Sometimes she seized on a recipe and if I suggested it was too complicated, she acted insulted. Then she went over what she needed to make this recipe, and I'd observe that she already had some of the ingredients. By the time we got to the market she asked, "Why do I have this on the list?"

"Well Poppy, maybe it's for some recipe."

"Well, why do I need this?"

"I don't know why."

"Well, we'll think about it later."

She had completely forgotten our previous discussion.

The man at the meat counter couldn't figure it out. We walked up and down and she asked questions. Endless questions. We went over every bit of meat – I could tell you about every piece of meat in the store.

"Maybe I should have steak?" she said.

"Maybe, I don't know," I replied. "What about this rack of lamb?"

"Definitely not," she'd say and push on.

In a few minutes, she'd come back and get the lamb. It had to be her idea.

It was best going to shops like Cobs Bread up on Bayview Ave., or that fish market just up the street where they had known her a long time and could see she was having trouble.

I was never certain what she might choose. She went in, looked around, and then left without saying a word. She had always been demanding. Now she had become ornery… ornery to the verge of causing serious trouble. When we went to Summerhill Market, I now stood behind her at the counter and used hand signals to alert the clerk to what we needed. She hauled out the glare if they offered unsolicited help, so I waved my hand to indicate they should stay away. Then I gestured to let them know it was OK to approach her, and nodded to indicate that she had decided on her choice. The clerks and I got a real system going. It was a bit of a joke, but I took pains to make sure Poppy never realized what was happening.

She sometimes wondered what was going on and the indication of that was a fierce glare and a hostile, "If I wanted your help I would ask for it."

I always tried my best to avoid setting her off. Once she went to the fridge and pulled out the mayonnaise: "We don't need corn – here it is."

"Yes, you're right, we don't need any corn," I said.

She got mixed up on what things were, but I felt there was no point in forcing her to recognize what she had done. That seemed unnecessarily upsetting and wouldn't have accomplished anything. I didn't want her to come back to reality too quickly. I would never ever put her on the spot.

One day Emma, in her wisdom, gave Poppy one of those yellow sticky notes and said, "This is important Poppy. Something you need to remember."

If the truth were told, at this point Poppy was remembering very little, although that didn't matter at all. She simply wouldn't accept anyone telling her what to do.

She handed the note back to Emma, who quickly thrust it back at her. Back and forth it went, back and forth, until Poppy finally seized it and plastered it on Emma's forehead.

I was getting concerned. Poppy had never hit anyone yet, but she had certainly come close, and this confrontation was quickly escalating to a new high (or low).

Emma didn't give up. She was determined to see this through. She pulled the sticky note off her forehead and demanded that Poppy take it. Poppy took it and again smacked it on top of Emma's head. Hard. "God damn it," she said. "I don't want it."

As she did this, I stepped between them and put my hands up. "OK ladies, end of round one."

I turned to Poppy, who seemed on the verge of throttling Emma. She stopped, looked me right in the eye, and then wilted. I stepped back.

Emma said. "Poppy, you shouldn't have done that."

Poppy only looked at us blankly. She had already moved on, forgetting the whole altercation.

Another time I was asked to introduce a new caregiver as a friend of mine. They thought that would smooth the waters a little. It certainly didn't. I felt somewhat dodgy about this new nurse – she seemed so sweet and nice, not Poppy's cup of tea at all. I suggested that she introduce herself as a maid. I suspected that Poppy would like the idea of a maid.

Unfortunately, few people want to be a maid, even a make-believe one.

We sat down and Poppy said, "What are you doing here?"

"I'm a nurse and I'm here to help you. I like helping elderly people."

Meghan, the new social worker, glanced at me and we both cringed. We could see that Poppy was ready to blow.

"Let's discuss it later," I said.

The nurse looked at Poppy and said, "I hope we meet again."

Poppy glared at her. "I hope not."

Afterwards Poppy launched into Meghan. "I don't need anyone but him." She pointed at me.

One incident was extremely telling. I reminded her that she probably needed cat food and offered to go and look. She said no, then seemed to pull back a little and said, "If you wouldn't mind."

Then finally, "Yes, good idea."

This seemed to me to be a new stage in her disease. Taking care of the cat food was of enormous personal importance to Poppy. To give it up really seemed to say a lot about her self-confidence. I suppose it also represented a major breakthrough in her willingness to trust me. It was hardly the kind of breakthrough I would want to cheer about, however.

One night, the caregiver called me at home to come down right away. She was panicky; she claimed the house was flooding. In truth, when I arrived, it was just a matter of finding the shutoff valve to the toilet, although it took a few minutes to discover where the valve was located. I didn't mind. There was a sense of excitement in Poppy's disasters. Of course, I wanted to help her. There was also a sense of being involved in something a little momentous – our own little emergencies, so to speak.

Poppy often put the wrong soap in the dishwasher, and the suds overflowed all over the kitchen. She blamed the caregivers. We marked the soap containers, but she still got them mixed up. We wanted to leave only one container there,

but she insisted on keeping both. This confusion happened
once or twice a week.

One day she insisted on making her own coffee and forgot to put the top on the grinder. Panic. Then of course, she couldn't move quickly enough to turn it off. There was coffee everywhere. I'm sure you can still find traces of it in the kitchen and even down the stairs. After that, there was always a delicious aroma of coffee in the kitchen. It was the day the coffee hit the fan.

Poppy usually used a credit card when she shopped. This caused trouble, as she could never remember her PIN number. Nevertheless, using cash was a nightmare. She always rummaged around trying to find her wallet and locate the right change. She'd spent long minutes counting out fifty-eight cents change instead of just giving the cashier a bill, while other customers and the salesperson looked on, shuffling their feet and rolling their eyes. Sometimes, she recognized their impatience and become frustrated and aggressive. That last summer she finally handed me the card and said, "Just do it."

Keeping the linen clean was another major challenge. The constant cycle of caregivers and Poppy's increasing incontinence meant that sheets needed washing frequently. At first, Poppy insisted on washing them at home, but this had to stop because she always put too much soap in the washer and the suds overflowed the machine. Eventually, Poppy and I loaded the bedding in the car and carried it up to the laundry service twice a week. There were lots of

134 sheets, piled high in the back of the station wagon. I suggested pick-up and delivery laundry service, but she insisted we take it ourselves. Poppy never faltered, she insisted on lugging the load to the cleaners from the car. Her laundry bill was staggering.

Poppy was feeding the caregivers, the dog, and the garbage can at this point; a third of the food hit the garbage. I felt sorry for the poor dog. Usually, his dinner included some butter tart, strudel, and carrots.

The caregivers tried to throw out Prince's unacceptable food, and replace it with fresh kibble, but this manoeuvre had to be handled very carefully. The same was true of cleaning out the fridge, when we found food at the back in dreadful condition. Poppy was completely unconcerned.

The caregivers always wanted to know when we were going out, so they could do chores that Poppy couldn't stand them doing. Then I'd phone to tell them we were coming back, so they weren't caught in the act.

Often during that last winter, Poppy quizzed me in detail as to the wind and temperature and so on. We then had a lengthy discussion about what coat to wear. After intently listening to my weather report and apparently accepting my word, she opened the door and went outside to see for herself.

One bitterly cold day, I convinced her to wear what had been her mother's full-length beaver coat. It almost touched the ground and had a big hood on it. It was a gorgeous coat

and looked good on Poppy, but I think she felt conspicuous    135
in it. She only wore it once.

\*\*\*

# Still Happy Moments

Even as these troubles surged around us, Poppy still surprised me with moments of happiness and lucidity. Many of her faculties were declining, but others would sometimes snap into dramatic focus.

I've always had trouble spelling and pronouncing 'croissant,' and Poppy, who could speak several languages, would make me say it over and over until I had pronounced it correctly. She demanded that I use the correct French accent, and as I struggled with it, she would scold me until I got it right. Then she fussed over my spelling.

'Strudel' was another. I didn't pronounce it with the proper German roll of the tongue, and Poppy insisted I keep trying until I got it right. She obviously had fun with this. She went down the shopping list and checked the spelling on everything. I suspect it was a bit of a daily escape for her. We were getting the same thing every day, but she still checked the spelling meticulously and insisted on testing my pronunciation.

A similar situation developed at the liquor store where we'd wander around looking at all the wines. Poppy really knew her wines, and again insisted on correcting my pronunciation of whatever we were considering. In the end, we always bought the Chardonnay. Keeping my sense of humour during these expeditions was a challenge.

She had regular calls from Anna and Mary Johnston and others, and when she was on the telephone, she spoke in a manner that was absolutely normal. She was a completely different person on the telephone. When I arrived, she was sometimes talking with someone and sounded fine. It was a peculiar quirk. If I had the chance to do it again, I would use the telephone a lot more in dealing with her.

Poppy was still physically strong. One day she asked if I minded lifting a buffet in the living room while she tucked a corner of the carpet under it. I couldn't budge it. She elbowed me out of the way, lifted the buffet, held it while I put the rug under it, and then let it down. I would have hated to be around if someone tried to steal her purse.

One spring day of that last year, I came to pick Poppy up and found her meeting with the gardener and his three student helpers. They were trimming the hedges at the front, and were dealing with some roses. Poppy launched into a detailed explanation of what she wanted. The gardener had brought in some new roses, and they were the wrong shade of pink – not exactly what Poppy had in mind.

The gardener and his assistants grew silent and listened in awe as Poppy explained the effect she was trying to achieve, and how the plants had to be just the right colour. In addition, they must be placed in just the right positions to produce the desired effect. She knew more than they did.

The episode in the garden was one of the last times I saw her take control of a situation and carry it off with absolute ease. She was straightforward and professional – a born leader. When one of the students asked a question, she calmly and logically provided the answer. It was so interesting to watch: Here was a woman whose short-term memory was so far gone that she was destined for a nursing home, yet her long-term memory about horticulture kicked in and she simply took over and ruled the day.

Poppy always maintained her interest in animals and birds. She had four bird feeders in the garden, and she could readily identify most of the little guys. Right up until the end, she and I often stood in the living room and watched the birds at the feeders and the birdbath. She obviously enjoyed this and was happy to stand there for a long time discussing the birds' antics. It was very poignant.

A neighbour complained about all the bird food everywhere. The feeders attracted squirrels, and Prince then would chase them over the fence into the neighbour's back yard. Poppy paid no attention to the complaint. Birds were more important to her than a few squirrels.

That spring we went to two operas, two ballets, and the Shaw Festival. Emma also arranged for the three of us to go to the Royal Ontario Museum to see Jane Goodall, the scientist who specialized in chimpanzees. At the last minute, Emma couldn't make it so Poppy and I went alone.

Poppy had been to Africa, and had donated to the Jane Goodall Foundation. We had perfect seats and she sat there enthralled, her face alight, completely mesmerized by Goodall's presentation. When we came out, I was pretty excited myself, and blurted out, "Wasn't that excellent?"

"Yes."

She never mentioned it again.

At the ballet she sat enraptured – soaking it all in. God forbid if any one sneezed or made a noise. She was so attentive and she hummed along with the music. How many people do you know who can hum along to the score from a ballet?

We sang singsongs on the way home. Singing was a short-term memory experience that made her very happy.

She still had a good sense of humour, though it became increasingly ribald. Once, she observed that I didn't swear around her. I hummed and hawed. I can swear as well as anyone, but I've never felt comfortable swearing in front of a woman. It's a generational thing I guess.

"Say shit," she said.

"Oh, no."

"You say shit," she insisted.

Finally, I blurted it out.

"Now that's better," she said.

This victory led to her reciting by heart a truly disgusting poem that she had learned in her school days. It seemed to contain every possible obscene and vulgar word in the English language. She was very keen on my learning it so I could pass it on to others. When I told her I didn't know anyone who I could tell it to, she laughed. Thankfully, she seemed to recognize the truth in that.

***

# The Caregivers

There is no point in denying reality. Despite moments when the clouds seemed to clear, the trend was there for all to see; and the trend was downward.

Nothing captured the nasty side of Poppy's predicament and personality more than her relationship with the caregivers. As I mentioned earlier, her family had brought in professional caregivers to support her as her problems became more obvious. Over time, this had increased from several days a week to, finally, full-time service.

The problem was that Poppy did not want these caregivers. She hated having strangers in her house, interfering with her way of doing things. She could not abide the notion that these people were there to help her, when she was adamant that she needed no help. Her insistence on independence made no sense of course, because she was getting worse, and her willingness to give up more and more of the decision-making to me and her children made it clear that she realized it. However, common-sense doesn't always prevail. She didn't want the caregivers and she resisted them in every way she could, as long as she could.

She yelled at them when they tried to do things for her. She reprimanded them when they answered the door or tried to help her with the cat. She refused to eat with them. She regularly inspected the fridge to see if their food was infringing on the space reserved for hers. When they worked in the kitchen, she watched over every move and criticized the way they did things.

She told them they had no conception of how to cook food, and she called one of the caregivers "Pinhead." She glared until it was easy to imagine her grabbing someone by the throat. She was a strong woman. It would take a brave individual to stand up to her threats for very long.

Poppy had a diabolical talent for spotting weakness. She couldn't stand weakness. There was one sweet little nurse who scurried around the house, terrified of Poppy but determined against all odds to help her lead a better life. She seemed willing to jump through hoops to assist Poppy, and Poppy simply put her through the grinder.

"Go away. I don't need you," or,

"I don't need that," or,

"I don't want you. Stay out of my way," or,

"I don't know why you're here."

The result, of course, was that there was a constant turnover of caregivers. They laughed off the first unpleasant encounters with Poppy, but after a few more insults, they refused to take it any longer. Off they'd go. Poppy made it so clear that they weren't wanted. Who could blame them for giving up when the messages were all so negative?

That's not to say that the caregivers were without blemish. They almost uniformly insisted on "helping" her. This, I had learned long before, was the last thing Poppy could abide. She abhorred accepting help. All of the caregivers tried to change her, or to get her to do things another way that in their minds was better for her. Their changes were probably for the better, but Poppy fought them off.

She seemed to feel, 'Why should I change? It's my home.'

I know that when it comes to feelings it's important to be discreet. Avoid arguments. Deal with people gently. Over and over, I saw these professional caregivers barge ahead with their ideas and their own agendas. They had little apparent recognition or appreciation of the impact their methods might be having on someone who was seeing her sanity and her whole way of life thrown into disarray.

Several times, I tried to tell them to move more slowly, to come at things more obliquely rather than a head-on confrontation – to try to go around the mountain rather than going straight through it. My suggestions seemed to affront their professionalism. They knew better. The result was anguish for everyone.

It probably didn't help, of course, that the caregivers saw me being treated differently from them. As the months went by, Poppy told me to just come in every morning and sit in the living room. Then I was to sit in the dining room. Then I was encouraged to sit and read the paper. Then I should have a coffee. This really bothered some of the caregivers, who didn't know who I was or my history with Poppy. They were carefully monitored regarding their coffee consumption, but here I was drinking it freely.

Finally, Poppy started laying out a beautiful Limoges cup and saucer for my coffee. It matched the walls of the dining room. She liked me or she liked men, but whatever it was, I was doing something she liked and the caregivers, in her mind, were doing the opposite. The message was clear to everyone.

Only two caregiver "guests" lasted until the end. They accomplished this by staying out of Poppy's way as much as possible. They each had a lovely room with a TV and a chair and a full private bathroom. They hid in there most of the day when Poppy was at home, emerging only to make dinner. This suited Poppy just fine.

***

# Planning The Exodus

Eventually, it became obvious that Poppy was becoming a danger to herself and others. A new arrangement was needed.

The kitchen had always been her domain, but now it was unsafe to let her prowl around as she had previously. For instance, she turned on the water tap, and then walked out of the room and forgot about it.

She occasionally left the gas on, and the smell filled the house, until either one of the caregivers or even a neighbour called the fire department. We tried to pacify the police officers and firefighters who became aware of her problem and did their best to treat it all sympathetically, but still had an essential job to do. There was little doubt that it was dangerous to leave her, even with 24-hour caregivers in attendance.

Emma decided to take the dials off the gas stove. Poppy blithely observed that the dials had been lost but said that didn't matter; she'd simply turned the switches by hand. She proceeded to do just that, much to everyone's chagrin.

The caregivers made an effort to keep an eye on her when she was in the kitchen, but of course, she resented the intrusion on her world and usually tried to send them packing.

Poppy lived in fear that her children would move her to the U.S. and put her in an institution. She often alluded to this, especially after one of her calls from Anna, who often, I gathered, would refer to some future time when Poppy would have to give up her home. I am sure Anna was simply trying to help her mother prepare for what lay ahead, but it would send Poppy into a panic.

One day I arrived just after she'd gotten off the phone with Edward or Anna. She said, "I don't like what I'm hearing."

"Poppy, no one is going to do anything without your complete consent. This is your house and you can stay in it until Hell freezes over."

"Are you sure?"

"Yes, Poppy. I've been there with other people. I've been there with other people in my family."

These could have been little lies, but I was trying to make her happy. She listened, asked a few questions, and seemed to feel relieved. I asked, "Poppy, what do you think your children will do?"

I think that question made her realize that I did have a point. Poppy was too smart to buy the whole package. She had always been convinced that in the end, they would trick her into leaving her home. She saw these telephone conversations as a prelude to war.

Anna often called to remind her of things to do like seeing the doctor or getting someone to go with her when she walked the dog. This would really get Poppy's dander up. It was innocent enough from Anna's point of view, but Poppy could recognize what lay behind it.

In February, Anna announced that she was coming to town.

"Anna is coming to see me. We're going to see some doctor. I don't like it."

"Well Poppy, at our age seeing a doctor is part of life," I replied.

Anna and Poppy met with the psychiatrist in March. Afterwards, Anna simply said that something had to be done. "We don't know how fast," she said to me. "But we'll let you know."

I think Anna and her brothers decided after the psychiatrist's appointment that Poppy had to move into a nursing home. It must have been a tough decision to make. Anna was not one for precipitous action. She knew how much Poppy loved her home and her independence. She certainly heard different tales about her mother's capabilities – or lack of them.

Several of the neighbours, as well as Emma, spoke to Anna opposing a move. They thought Poppy was still doing well enough, and with more intensive care could stay in her home for a bit longer. Behind her back, there were the predictable comments that Anna wasn't doing enough for her mother, and wanted her in a home so she wouldn't have to bother with her as much. However, the neighbours weren't seeing what the caregivers and Emma and I were seeing on a daily basis. I could appreciate that the family was planning ahead. It takes time for such things to happen. They wanted to avoid a spur-of-the-moment decision that might leave Poppy in a less than desirable position.

Anna listened to everyone and I could see she was struggling to be as fair as possible; to listen with an open mind. I could also see she was in a fix. Sure, they could delay the move, but that would likely only make it more painful and more difficult when it actually had to happen. Doing it a little sooner rather than after a crisis, they could at least try to manage the transition better.

A month later, in April, Anna met with Emma and me in the kitchen, to announce the family's decision: Poppy would leave in August. She would be moving to an upscale nursing home near Hartford that had plenty of experience dealing with patients suffering from dementia. As most people know, you can't just plan to place someone in a home and expect instant admission. You must plan months in advance. Anna and Edward had found a beautiful place in Plymouth right on the ocean. They had paid to hold it empty while they managed the departure from Toronto.

Their plan was to invite Poppy to a weekend visit with Edward in Hartford, and once she was there, he would announce that he had unexpected company coming for a few

days, and they were going to have her stay in another place
for a while. The assumption was that once she was in the
new place, the staff would take charge of shifting her into a
long-term state of mind.

Anna asked me if I would mind flying to Hartford with
Poppy. They thought it would be too suspicious if one of
them went with her. Poppy had always feared a day like this,
and their presence might just trigger a reaction that would
snooker their plans.

I was flattered, of course, that they would trust me with
this kind of task. I suppose they could see that Poppy and I
had bonded so well over the months, and that I was the one
she would most trust to escort her on her "long weekend in
Hartford." In fact, I was the only one she would accept as her
travelling companion.

That night I talked it over with Stephanie.

"I'd be furious if you did that to me," she said.

"But this is different. She's literally losing her mind. And
her family is so far away."

"I'd still be furious. I think I'd be most furious at you.
You're her best friend."

"I know, but sometimes a real friend has to do unpleasant things in order to protect his friend."

Stephanie paused and looked around the room. She took
a deep breath. "Well OK, but how are you going to feel when
this is all over? Will you be able to look at yourself in the
mirror and not feel guilty?"

It was my turn to pause and think. Stephanie was making some good points. I didn't want to regret this the rest of my life. "I'm going to keep my options open," I said. "I'll tell Anna I'll do it, but if I change my mind…well, I'll just change my mind."

Anna was extraordinarily considerate of me in her planning. Once I had agreed, she said that if the date was inconvenient for me, they would change it to suit my needs. I was free. In as much as I regretted seeing Poppy lose her home this way, I at least wanted to do everything in my power to make sure the journey was as painless as possible.

Secrecy was the big issue. The 'transfer' had to be well planned. We all knew that Poppy would never leave if she knew what was really going to happen. Nobody liked the secrecy, but there was no viable alternative.

We hunkered down to lead as normal a life as possible for the next few months until the transition finally happened, trying at all costs not to alert Poppy to what lay ahead.

I hated the thought of her leaving her home and I empathized with Emma in wishing she could be kept longer if given more intensive care. Realistically, I could see that this really wouldn't have achieved a great deal. A move was inevitable. Poppy clearly over-estimated her ability to lead her life – she would eventually kill herself in the kitchen or go for a walk and never come home.

It had to be done.

Soon.

Whether it was done in June, August, or October really 153
didn't matter. Delaying would be simply putting off the inevitable, and running an increasing risk of something terrible
happening either to Poppy or to one of the caregivers.

The idea of more intensive care made sense on the
surface, but the fact was that the caregivers were actually
giving her less care rather than more. They were literally
hiding in their rooms for a lot of the time. They were scared
of her. They wouldn't come out unless they had to. She didn't
want them.

"What are they doing here?" she asked repeatedly. "Stay
out of my way!" she barked.

She often told me how upsetting it was to have strangers
in her house, and she wanted to know if I knew why they
were there. Did I know what was going on, she asked.

One day, one of the caregivers took the initiative to clean
up the cat litter in Poppy's room and Poppy was furious. The
expletives flew. Under no circumstances was anybody to do
any such thing. The cat was her responsibility and she was
quite capable of looking after it. Don't do it again!

Poppy's anger (and the infamous wrathful glare) was
aimed at a sweet woman who was really just trying to help
her. You could imagine how the poor woman felt. Poppy,
despite her slender frame was a muscular and powerful
woman. No one doubted that she could do a lot of damage
in a short time if her rage got away from her.

In the kitchen, the caregivers tried to cook her meat, and
she pushed them out of the way. She told them she cooked

154    her own meat. They always overcooked it. She wanted it rare.
One day, grabbing a hunk of raw meat in her hand, she tore
off a chunk with her teeth and chewed on it angrily. "That's
how I want it," she said. "Blood rare. That's how I like it."

God bless Emma. She had the right personality. Poppy
really ranted at her, and Emma just accepted it. Emma rarely
took Poppy's attacks personally. But sometimes she started
crying and then Poppy backed off a little and said, "Oh,
don't worry."

Poppy seemed to realize that Emma was special. She
tolerated Emma. She didn't want the others. Well, she didn't
want Emma either, but she seemed to understand that she
needed her.

Early in May, Poppy came down the stairs with her
hands full of clumped cat litter. She said, "I'll take it down
myself in my hands."

I knew then that it was time. She was increasingly incon-
tinent and had lost interest in keeping herself clean. The
caregivers told me she stepped into the shower and stepped
right out again, barely wet. Her feet desperately needed a
pedicure but she resisted the suggestion.

The situation worsened and she sometimes appeared
with a wet spot on the back of her pants. I'd say, "Poppy,
you must have sat on something while you were in the park
with Prince."

She'd immediately go up and change. It became a signal
between her and me. It broke my heart, but I knew what I

had to do. Feeling about Poppy as I did, I resolved to carry it off as best I could.

***

# Flying To Hartford

Our last day had arrived; it was a Tuesday – a beautiful, sunny day, but I woke up worried. The carefully-wrought plan made sense, but so many things could go wrong. Getting Poppy through the various hoops of flying to Hartford seemed daunting enough, but there was the worry that she would discover what I was really up to, and that would lead who knows where?

In addition, I was saying goodbye. To Poppy, I was saying goodbye for a long weekend before we would be reunited. To me, it was goodbye. Period. The last goodbye. I felt disloyal.

Despite all the careful planning, there was so much that could go wrong. I couldn't help thinking of that very first interview, when Poppy was just another challenge, and Prince had intervened to give me the edge I needed to enter her life. Now, a year and a half later, we had formed a bond that seemed special to both of us.

In my mind, Poppy and I had become a couple. Not a romantic couple, of course – there had never been anything like that in our relationship. However, we'd become very dependent on each other: She needed me. As her ability to control her own life slipped away from her, she had come to lean on me as the one person who could be relied on to respect her independence, and yet provide the gentle leadership her condition seemed to demand. Not that she would ever admit it, of course. Poppy was Poppy right to the end. I knew my place.

Now I was taking her, unbeknownst to her, on our last outing. Of course, it was for her own good. It was all very reasonable. She was going to be much better off in her new quarters. It was eminently sensible to have her well positioned in a secure environment. She would be close to her children before this terrible disease wreaked its final havoc. Nevertheless, I still felt like a traitor. A traitor who had better get going on his final assignment.

I got to the house around nine a.m., expecting Poppy to be ready. When I walked in the front door, it seemed like all hell was breaking loose.

"How dare the cleaning lady pack my clothes?" Poppy shouted.

She had that fearsome glare. Emma and two neighbours, Prince and I were all crowded into the vestibule, watching anxiously as Poppy ripped open her bag and started to pull out her clothes. "How can the cleaning lady know what I'm going to wear?" she demanded. "Now I have to start all over again and pick out what I really need. This is really too much."

"Now Poppy, you understand," said Emma, obviously quite unsure that anything was understandable. Desperate though I was to get started, I couldn't help thinking that Poppy was right. It scared me a little. We were skilfully stealing her away from her beloved home to a completely new existence because she wasn't capable of taking care of herself. She was clever enough to recognize that if she were going away for a short trip, then she didn't need all this clothing. This was a conflict, which set my antennae quivering anew.

"Now Poppy," said Emma. "This is just a little mistake, and we can fix it easily."

Poppy wasn't having any of that.

"I don't need the cleaning lady packing for me. And that's final."

"Good morning, Poppy," I said.

"Good morning." For a moment, she seemed to calm down and then just as quickly turned back to her bag.

"Poppy, we don't have time to repack," I said. "If we don't catch this flight your son may not be able to meet us."

That distracted her for a moment. Then another long-time neighbour popped through the door, hiding her real feelings about the whole charade in a display of gleeful bonhomie. "Oh Poppy," she said, "You're going to have such a wonderful time."

Poppy glanced at her, attempted a smile, and then turned back to the bag. "How dare these people do my packing for me?"

"Now listen, Poppy," said Emma.

Poppy either didn't hear her or decided to ignore her. The clothes continued to fly.

By now, I was getting desperate. I wasn't planning to let this incident screw up this mission.

"Poppy," I said. "Your son is waiting. If we miss this flight then we're really in trouble."

This time it caught. She dropped the bag, glared at me and said, "So let's get going."

The crisis was over, gone as quickly as it had surfaced. Emma stuffed the clothes back into Poppy's bag, and we silently shuffled out the door. Poppy turned to Prince and patted him on the head.

"Be a good boy," she said, "I'll see you next week."

Poppy marched right out and into Emma's car, assuming the front passenger seat, with me in the back. I glanced at my watch and calculated how much time we had wasted. All the ladies crowded round, wishing Poppy well. They were full of enthusiasm, hiding their real emotions at this final goodbye; but also, I am sure, determined to protect Poppy from the truth.

We drove down the driveway and pulled away; Poppy staring grimly down the road, apparently oblivious to the fact that she would never pass this way again. So I tell myself.

"We'd better move it along," I muttered. Emma took
heed. We sped through the traffic, Emma talking continu-
ously, anxious I am sure, to keep Poppy's mind off any sus-
picion that this trip was not entirely as advertised. Poppy, of
course, ignored all this and continued to stare down the road.

Emma let us off at the airport terminal and jumped out
to hug Poppy one last time. "Oh Poppy," she said, "have a
great weekend."

"See you next week," said Poppy.

"Poppy, let's not dawdle," I said.

"I don't dawdle."

Poppy was in such a nasty mood that I knew if someone
said anything in the least bit offensive to her, she would give
them what for. Not the ideal strategy when dealing with
airline people these days. We sailed through the formalities
without incident, walked quickly down through the departure lounge, and into the narrow gangway leading to the
airplane. Ahead, I could see the attendant standing by the
door, her hand poised to slam it shut.

Then a last-second mishap: Poppy had mislaid her
boarding pass. It was in that huge, black purse of hers – a
bottomless pit that seemed to gobble up everything she
dropped into it, never to be seen again. Poppy dove in
gamely, determined to find it.

I turned to the attendant. "We may have to hold the
plane a couple of minutes while we straighten this out."

Her answer was clear. "We don't hold the plane
for anyone."

Well, that was helpful.

Fortunately, Poppy came up with the pass and we rushed on, the door slamming shut behind us.

Poppy went on ahead down the narrow aisle, and I took advantage of the moment to lean over to the front cabin attendant. "Bear with me, please, if anything goes awry; this lady has Alzheimer's. She can be difficult."

The attendant smiled. "I understand. Thank you for telling me."

As we took off, I could see Emma's car down in the middle of the parking lot. God bless her, she had stayed on guard for us until the very last second. I mentioned it to Poppy, and she ventured a quick smile but didn't say anything. I could tell she was still in a funk.

Once in the air we were served wine and sandwiches. Poppy chose white I allowed myself a glass of red.

"This wine is terrible," Poppy announced after drinking half her glass.

"Poppy, let's trade," I said. "Maybe you'll like the red better."

She drank my red and announced that it wasn't much better. Then she declared the sandwiches inadequate, and I offered her mine. She found them not up to her standards, however she ate them.

It wasn't a long flight, an hour and a half. Neither of us had much to say. Poppy spent her time looking out the window. I imagined that she was reminiscing. Who knows what was going through her mind? She knew the area and had gone to school in some of the places over which we were flying.

"There's Buffalo," she said.

"Interesting."

"There's the Erie Canal."

"Well Poppy," I said. "That reminds me of that song you like: Fifteen years on the Erie Canal,

Had a great boss and had a great pal."

This was a song she used to enjoy, and suddenly reminded of it, she started singing it. Not so loud that anyone could hear, but she sang it through once and then hummed it quietly for quite a while. It must have brought back pleasant memories, because she seemed to relax a little.

There was one more near-crisis on the plane. About thirty minutes into the flight, Poppy took notice of a casually dressed man up ahead in the second row, who was chewing gum. I doubt I would have noticed him myself, but Poppy zeroed in on him. He must have loved his gum, for he had stuffed a great whack of it into his mouth, and was relentlessly and noisily chewing the living daylights out of it. Poppy took it upon herself to announce in a loud clear voice, "Isn't that disgusting? How could he be so rude?"

I nodded at her, hoping she would let it go. However, being Poppy, there was no chance of that. She kept repeating herself over and over for at least ten minutes, with my anxiety growing by the moment. Anyone close to us must have heard her, but fortunately, she never actually mentioned the word gum, so it was hard to connect her reprimand with anyone in particular.

I was grateful when the attendant finally made an announcement about immigration procedures in Hartford, and Poppy forgot the whole episode. This was a relief, because if the guy had ever confronted her, I know Poppy would have loved to take him on.

In the back of my mind, I was still convinced that Poppy could smell a rat. She had always been leery of these kinds of trips away from her home, and she had long suspected that one of these days her children would try to spirit her off. She much preferred them to visit her, and have less control over her. Whether this trip posed a real danger in her mind I will never know, but I mentioned Edward several times during the flight, and that seemed to keep her focused on the future rather than the threat.

By the time we landed, she was in a better mood. There was a vague smile on her face, and I could tell she was looking forward to seeing Edward.

\*\*\*

# A Smile At Twilight

We went through customs without trouble. Fortunately, they didn't check my carry-on, which was full of Poppy's clothing. Edward and Pamela, his partner, met us at the gate, looking suitably casual, and waving as if the queen had arrived. There were hugs and handshakes all around. Poppy didn't say much, and I wondered if her old fears of walking into a trap might be on her mind. As we walked down the corridor, she put her arm in Edward's, and looked up at him tenderly.

Pamela and I introduced ourselves and followed along behind. She asked me how the trip had gone, and I shrugged. "Nothing drastic, but it had its moments."

I explained to Pamela that my bag was in fact Poppy's, and that she needed to take it over without alerting Poppy. She nodded, and indeed that's what she later did.

Edward led us to a nice-looking Mexican restaurant just down the hall from the gate. It didn't take long to eat, and Poppy spent the majority of the time talking with Edward. I talked with Pamela.

Overhearing Poppy and Edward talk about the weekend and all the things he had planned for her, I couldn't help thinking how totally different she was with her son. This was the Catch 22 of the situation. If you had been at the next table, nothing would have appeared unusual. Keep in mind that she was healthy physically.

When we came to the door, Poppy and I looked at each other.

"See you next week," I said.

We shook hands, then suddenly she leaned forward, hugged me, and gave me a kiss. It was the most affection we had ever shared. The cynic in me says she was almost too affectionate for someone she was supposedly going to see again in three or four days. She stepped back and smiled. A warm and generous smile. The poet in me says it was a smile at twilight.

There was finality on both sides – some from her, some from me. I was sure she knew the truth.

"Have a great time, Poppy," I said, and turned to flee down the hall. I was still worried that she would grasp the enormity of the moment and it would escalate into something we would all regret.

At the end of the hall, I peeked around and saw them as they walked out the exit. Poppy didn't look back. Why would she? She didn't seem to be drawing a conclusion. She was concerned about Edward, not me. Rightly so. Thank goodness.

*Does she know?* I asked myself.

I couldn't help thinking that she was just too bright and too smart to let them get away with this. If I knew Poppy, she was thinking, "If they feel they can pull this over on me, they're wrong. I've been trapped before, and I know how to escape."

I walked over to the departures lounge and checked in for the flight back to Toronto. Flying home, I felt sad. We had deceived her, but there was no alternative. It felt like I had gone to someone's funeral, but no one had died. The family didn't want anyone from Toronto contacting her; they thought (probably rightly) that stirring up past memories would only confuse her. The cleaner the break the better. So be it.

I declined a drink on the way back, but I had a couple of stiff ones when I got home. The next morning when I woke up, I found myself reminding myself to make that familiar morning call. Nine-thirty came and went. Of course, I didn't call. Neither did Poppy.

Poppy was gone.

\*\*\*

# What Happened Then?

I have heard that Edward and Anna took Poppy on a merry chase for several days, visiting a slew of famous Hartford sites that she had long admired. Then, Friday afternoon, they settled her into a room in the nursing home. It was only for a night or two, they told her, a temporary measure, because Edward had guests coming and needed the space at home. Soon she'd be back to his place.

That night, the nurses caught her walking down the driveway with her suitcase. Two nights later, she tried it again. They put her in lockdown. She was livid. Then, after Anna returned to her home in Utica, Poppy made several more breaks for freedom.

Edward called me and told me about how poorly Poppy was adjusting to the new place. I reminded him that Poppy had always read the newspaper in the morning, and that she had seemed to be most comfortable in her chaotic office. I suggested that if they arranged for *The New York Times* with her breakfast and allowed her room to become a little messy, she might feel more at home. Letting the housekeepers maintain her room spotlessly clean would only remind her that she was in a foreign environment. Edward thought this was a terrific idea, and told me later that they had done this and it certainly helped.

I heard that over several months Poppy gradually adjusted. As I write this, I have the impression that she has become relatively comfortable with her situation. She's forgotten her life in Toronto, and now appears to be content in her new home. This, I guess, is a roundabout way to say that she's continuing to go downhill mentally, but is being well taken care of and seems comfortable in her more sheltered situation. Apparently, she uses her time trying to teach French to her new friends. Sometimes I picture her haranguing some innocent old gentleman to pronounce "croissant" correctly. Good luck to her and him.

Emma was already close to perfection in my mind, but after Poppy left she escalated her efforts and became a volunteer caregiver for a nursing home on Yonge St. I am sure she is just as competent with her new clients as she was with Poppy, and as accommodating with any social workers she might encounter. Almost as importantly, Emma stepped in and agreed to take care of Samantha, the cat.

Anna gave Prince to a retired policeman who had previously owned a Doberman. I still see them walking the streets every so often. I purposely avoid encountering them. I don't know why. Well I guess I do. Why stir up old memories?

Anna and Edward continue to spend a lot of time with Poppy, and call me every so often to fill me in on her situation. They did the right thing for her. They continue to do the right thing.

So what did I learn from all this that might be of help to someone else in a similar situation? Everyone is different, of course, and what worked for me won't necessarily work for others. You have to try your best, be flexible and sensitive, and then adjust based on what you learn.

I hope I have conveyed to you the importance, even in the worst of times, of allowing a person with dementia as much scope as is safely possible to set their own direction. Avoid a 'helping' kind of attitude; instead, try to focus on suggestions and ideas to motivate the person to make their own decisions, or at least to feel comfortable with decisions made around them.

Try to avoid forcing decisions on them. It may seem to you that pushing a person to make a decision helps them maintain their freedom and individuality. I found that at times even a minor decision would sometimes confuse Poppy and trigger frustration, which in turn led to anger and depression.

Similarly, I don't know if I would ask many questions of a person suffering from some form of dementia. From my experience, even asking a question like, "Isn't it a nice day?" or "Are you happy?" seemed to put pressure on Poppy. Once a person has lost a lot of memory, it's very difficult to make a decision, even a simple one. Decisions seem to trigger emotions and memories, perhaps of things they'd prefer to forget, perhaps of things they've already forgotten and are now sad to be reminded of because of what they've lost. Again, it's a matter of tailoring the approach to the individual situation.

Perhaps the personality becomes exaggerated in a situation like this. A person with dementia lives with a constant degree of frustration. He or she knows something is wrong, but can't put his or her finger on it. This causes a once-calm personality to become inflamed.

I'd also avoid getting upset over any errors they make. What's the point? Does it really matter in the end if they look at a picture of you and say it's your brother or sister? So what if they forget the day of the week? Think of it – in their world, there probably aren't many reasons to distinguish between the days of the week. What the heck...there are plenty of caregivers there who will remember for them. Don't bother about it. Making an issue of it will only trigger bad feelings.

It is important to build on the patient's personal habits. I found that if I suggested corn, for example, Poppy would want peas. Her automatic reaction was to do the opposite of what I proposed. I learned over time that when peas were available, then I would propose corn. She would choose peas and both of us would be content.

Sometimes it's helpful to try planting a small seed in their minds, hoping it may take root and grow. "Poppy, let's go for a drive later," just may elicit an 'OK,' either now or later.

173

My main lesson is to roll with the punches. Let the person live in his or her world, rather than trying to draw them back into the world they've lost. Keep the conversation as upbeat and happy as you can. The more serious you get, the more upsetting it is for a person with Alzheimer's. If I had to sum it all up in one little phrase, I would say, "Keep life gentle and easy."

I look back on my time with Poppy as one of the most memorable and satisfying periods of my life. Poppy showed me what it takes to set your own path in life and stick to it, come hell or high water. She may have driven the rest of us crazy but she knew what she wanted and she went after it, full speed ahead.

She had a good life. Yes, tragedy struck, but I don't think she saw it that way at all. When I heard her talking on the phone, I suspect I was hearing more of the former Poppy than I ever saw in my daily interactions with her. She seemed elated, engaged, fully on her game. Occasionally, when she met an old friend in the street or at the market, they laughed, hugged, and carried on as if they were old school chums who hadn't seen each other in years. She didn't know who he or she was, of course, but that didn't matter. She was alive and full of fun.

At most other times, though, I sensed she was consciously trying to keep her emotions under control. We went to see *My Fair Lady* and she loved it; but it was a controlled enthusiasm rather than a spirit of unbridled elation. I suspect that had something to do with her disease. I don't think she had been so restrained before her illness. Now, however, she knew something was wrong; something beyond her understanding; something weighing on her all the time.

By the time Poppy and I said our final goodbyes, there was a sadness in her life and demeanour, which hadn't been there when I first met her. In the beginning, she was a positive force, despite her looming fate. She knew what she wanted and she was determined to get it. However, near the end, I think she was no longer sure of what she wanted. I could see the gloom creep into her life.

Even at the worst of times there was little complaining or self-pity or hiding in a corner, afraid of the world. To the best of her ability, Poppy grabbed hold of each day as it came, drawing as much pleasure and achievement from it as she could. She never lowered her head to anyone. In the worst of times, when fate seemed to have dealt her a monstrous blow and circumstances seemed preordained to make that blow even worse, Poppy would not back off in her efforts to maintain her independence and her dignity.

She was an eccentric, yes. In some ways, she was a spoiled brat. She had her opinions, and heaven help the unsuspecting do-gooder who blundered into her way. She could occasionally be a tyrant; a bull in a china shop. Her friendship and trust were hard to gain.

Nevertheless, I shall always remember those magic moments when Poppy and I clicked. We started as incorrigible opposites and ended up a happy pair. We never argued; if there was a difference of opinion it was usually very subtle, and unless it was obviously off the wall, we just did what she wanted.

My life with Poppy was an incredible experience. I grew to think the world of her. She was one hell of a person. If you had seen us together, you would have asked, "How do they ever get along?" Yet we knew each other's likes and dislikes, and our limitations.

It was sad that we were getting to know each other so well and yet were doomed to part. As I took over more and more of her decisions, I think her feelings towards me grew. She realized that she was better off with me than without. I'm human – I enjoy being needed.

I looked forward to each day with her. Few days were straightforward. Our time together was intense, but rarely unpleasant. It was like going to a first-rate hockey game or a gripping play. There was always something interesting on the horizon. From minute to minute, I never knew what was going to happen next.

Poppy was a woman with a mission. She liked getting out and seeing things at her own pace. The domestic trials and disasters were all part of the challenge; although I suppose that at the time I was probably more than a little perturbed by some of her antics.

Still, looking back, I can only chuckle and wish she were still here, still telling me where to turn, where to park, and how to choose the best veggies and fish for dinner.

I took a short break after Poppy went to Hartford and then returned to work for the agency. I began looking after an elderly man who couldn't be left alone for a second, but could not interact with anyone, including me. It wasn't very challenging, and I left that assignment soon after it began.

Everyone has to move on at some time or another, and that's exactly what I am doing. My grandsons, cars, and playing chess are back in the spotlight. The future lies ahead and it is a wondrous thing – I am grateful to be here to savour it. I am buoyed along by the memories of my fine adventures with Poppy. I take a hefty measure of her courage and energy with me as I trundle on down the road.

# Robert Loyst

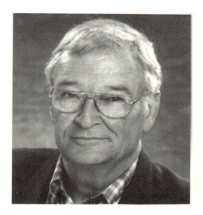

Native Torontonian Robert Loyst travelled internationally during his career as a sales executive. Upon retirement, he missed being busy, so he took a job as an aide to Poppy, an elderly woman in the first stages of Alzheimer's. An avid reader, Robert understood that his unique, unexpected experiences with Poppy were tailor-made for a book. Robert and his wife Stephanie live in Toronto with their cat, Squish.

# Wayne Yetman

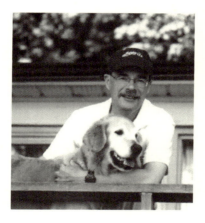

Wayne Yetman's non-fiction has been published in many magazines and newspapers, including the Reader's Digest. His fiction has appeared in *The Antigonish Review*, *The New Quarterly* and *The Fiddlehead* among others. When Robert shared tales of his experiences with Poppy, Wayne too saw a wonderful book and partnered up with Robert to tell Poppy's story.

Printed in Canada